NUMERACY
IN CHILDREN'S
NURSING

NUMERACY IN CHILDREN'S NURSING

Arija Parker

Senior Lecturer
School of Health
University of Central Lancashire (UCLAN)

WILEY Blackwell

Library of Congress Cataloging-in-Publication Data is available on request
9780470658390

A catalogue record for this book is available from the British Library.

Wiley also publishes its books in a variety of electronic formats. Some content that appears in print may not be available in electronic books.

Cover image courtesy of Biruta Daina Jefimovs

Set in 9/12pt Trade Gothic LT Std by Aptara Inc., New Delhi, India
Printed and bound in Malaysia by Vivar Printing Sdn Bhd

1   2015

Contents

CONTRIBUTORS   vi

ACKNOWLEDGEMENTS   vii

ABOUT THE COMPANION WEBSITE   ix

GETTING STARTED: HOW TO USE THIS BOOK   x

1   THE ROLE OF NUMERACY IN NURSING AND HEALTHCARE PRACTICE   1

2   COUNTING AND MEASURING   27

3   BASIC NUMERACY SKILLS UNDERPINNING CHILDREN AND YOUNG PEOPLE'S NURSING PRACTICE   65

4   ADVANCING ONWARDS: TAKING THE WHOLE NUMBER APART   97

5   PUTTING THE PIECES TOGETHER – A FORMULA FOR CHILDREN'S NURSES   131

6   ADMINISTERING MEDICINES AND MANAGING NUMBERS IN MORE COMPLEX SETTINGS – THE
     PHARMACIST AND NEONATAL NURSING PERSPECTIVES   161
     Gerard Donaghy and Lisa McCormack

7   CHILD DEVELOPMENT AND NUMBER SENSE   191

8   WHERE DO I GO FROM HERE?   221

ANSWERS   227

APPENDIX: FAMOUS MATHEMATICIANS   237

REFERENCES AND BIBLIOGRAPHY   241

INDEX   247

Contributors

Gerard Donaghy
Neonatal Intensive Care Unit
Royal Preston Hospital
Preston, UK

Lisa McCormack
Neonatal Intensive Care Unit
Royal Preston Hospital
Preston, UK

Acknowledgements

Thank you to the nursing staff and pharmacists from the children's wards and neonatal unit at Royal Preston Hospital for their time and suggestions for case scenarios, and to all the children and families who have contributed their experiences to ensure that this book has a 'real' focus (even though their anonymity and confidentiality has been protected throughout as per NMC (2015) The Code). A big special thank you goes to Lisa and Gerard who have contributed a chapter to this book, thus ensuring that the 'specialist' neonatal perspective to more complex calculation is evident.

A special thank you goes to Elaine MacDonald and the team of diabetes specialist nurses she works with, for her input and expertise in relation to the management of children and young people with diabetes.

Thank you to the publishers for giving me this opportunity to develop a numeracy text book that is a little bit different from the usual that is with the focus on children and the unique addition of illustrations that I have to thank my sister, Biruta Daina Jefimovs, for. I thank all the people around her who have inspired her also – it is amazing how a visual image can generate so many thoughts and ideas which have added to the quality of the written work in this book.

Thank you for the help and support offered by my family who were both tested from a numeracy perspective (in addition to having to do the usual KS2 and KS3 homework) as well as having a mother/wife who became obsessed with numbers in general and so did not attend to her other duties with as much enthusiasm and passion as expected.

Thank you to many mathematicians, many of whom I did not know existed before starting to research this book – this appreciation of the world of numbers will no doubt continue to grow beyond the publication of this book to infinity and beyond (to quote Lightyear, B).

Thanks finally to all the writers of books and resources that support and inform the good numeracy practice in relation to nursing education that underpins this book.

Arija Parker

DISCLAIMER

Every attempt has been made to ensure that an up-to-date evidence base has been utilised when offering additional information and discussing the care of children, whose case scenarios form the basis for numeracy-related activities, though some artistic licence has been taken to illustrate the numeracy points being made to ensure that the learning in relation to numeracy is reinforced. So please do not rely totally on the brief information offered and read in greater depth than is offered here in relation to anatomy, physiology, pathophysiology and evidence-based practice.

In the same way some recognised nursing assessment tools such as PEWS and pain assessment charts, tools have been adapted to suit the needs of the fictitious hospital used in this book which are not tools that are in existence though have been developed from real life examples and references/bibliography included at the end of the book thus acknowledging the primary sources used.

About the companion website

Do not forget to visit the companion website for this book:

 www.wiley.com/go/parker/numeracy

There you will find valuable material designed to enhance your learning, including:

- Further information on some of the case scenarios in the book

- Numeracy activities and worksheets

- PowerPoints on addition, subtraction, multiplication and division

- Further resources including links to useful websites

- Templated materials to support your learning

Scan this QR code to visit the companion website

GETTING STARTED: HOW TO USE THIS BOOK

What you need to do and how to use this book

What do you need to give to this book? An open mind, a willingness to challenge some of the assumptions that you have about the world of mathematics and, as a result, change some of the ways you use mathematical skills in your nursing practice. What you will not need is a typical school mathematics toolkit that includes a ruler, protractor and compass.

What is included in this 'getting started' section is a numeracy toolkit that consists of this book and the accompanying website or Online Numeracy Experience (ONE) resource. The guidance that follows will help you navigate your way through the content and use the book and website to their best advantage.

Chapter layout

Each chapter follows a standard layout to ease navigation through the book, and all practice-related information is based on a fictional hospital called Arch Mede Hospital, a general hospital that caters for the health needs of children, as well as the adult population, of a city called Pythagoras and its surrounding areas. Because this is a children's nursing book, this allows us to view numeracy through the eyes and experiences of child patients, so illustrations, featuring Staff Nurse Dee Vision, appear throughout the book guiding you on your progress and journey through this nursing-focused numeracy adventure.

The children's wards at Arch Mede Hospital

- Alpha Ward 1 (The Neonatal Unit)
- Beta Ward 2 (The Children's Unit)
- Gamma Ward 3 (The Children's Day Case Surgery Unit)

The child, young person and family stories utilised are all based on real-life case studies taken from clinical practice areas and, in line with 'The Code' as NMC (2015) guidance, confidentiality and anonymity is protected throughout. The practice situations cover the most usual seen in most children's wards in District General Hospitals throughout the United Kingdom and are utilised to illustrate the numeracy skills being learned in the related chapter.

Learning focus and learning outcomes

These appear at the beginning of each chapter, followed by an outline of the case scenario.

Case scenario

Case scenarios include a basic outline of the child and family who are the focus of the numeracy activities for the relevant chapter. Some families will be referred to in other chapters also, although this will be clearly indicated for those of you who want to dip in and out of the book rather than work your way through the whole book. Not all the numerical data will be included in all the scenarios, although examples of most will appear in the case scenario files on the website ONE to allow you to set up your own numeracy problems and develop skills using all the examples included. The nursing and clinical information offered in each section and to each scenario relates to the numeracy issues under discussion in that chapter. The data included in the book and online will include examples of charts, that is, observation chart (including paediatric early warning score (PEWS)), fluid balance charts, blood results (if applicable), personal record books/diaries and other useful information. The core essential information will appear in the book whilst the remainder, such as charts, will appear on the website related to some of the children, young people and family who feature in the book.

The surnames used for children and family members are based on famous mathematicians – see the Appendix at the end of the book if you would like to find out more about the history of these amazingly intelligent and creative people.

Numeracy information

In each chapter the case scenario is followed by an introduction to the numeracy skills on which the chapter focuses; this is then followed by some numeracy activities to aid your understanding and learning. Each aspect of the numeracy activity will be explained in detail using worked examples. PowerPoint presentations supplement these text-based explanations on the website ONE with the intention that if one explanation does not aid your learning then the other should. The book is designed to take a sequential approach by starting with the basics, thus building the learning from bottom to top, brick-by-brick. This should ensure that you are able to start from the beginning and get to the end successfully learning in a logical and progressive manner. Answers for the numeracy activities appear at the end of each chapter.

The companion website ONE

Chapters are designed to be short, user friendly and accessible. As a result, further numeracy activities and worksheets are placed on the website (ONE) which supports this book. Here you can find more activities to help you continue to practise, as well as links to other numeracy-related materials and websites, both generic and nursing based.

You can also print off useful resources such as squared paper, multiplication lattices and games/activities to use with the children you care for as well as many other things. Whilst working through the book it will be useful to have easy access to the ONE resource to further practise your skills from the individual sections of the book. You will be guided to access these resources where you see this icon.

Websites and other useful resources and information

There are many additional useful textbooks, websites and online resources that will supplement your learning; these are included as links on the ONE resource and within the chapters also. These will be identified using the same computer icon as the ONE resource.

Nursing children and young people and numeracy-related hints and tips!

The very practical nature of this book allows for practice-related useful information to be added as you journey through each chapter and is indicated by the following icon.

Practise your numeracy skills

Throughout the book there are opportunities to practise numeracy skills following worked examples that precede them, shown by this icon.

The answers are included at the end of each chapter.

Personal development through numeracy-related learning

All chapters will offer advice on how to utilise your learning to develop personal and professional practice. Should you choose to do this it will help you meet Post-registration education and practice (PREP) requirements as well as help build your professional portfolio (NMC, 2007). This is indicated by the following icon.

A blank template for reflection on numeracy practice is included in Section 5 of the ONE resource and a completed one is shown below and follows a reflective cycle that is adapted from pre-existing reflective models ((Gibbs, 1988; Johns, 2004) with a particular focus on the work of Moon (1999)) and includes a section that asks you to identify numeracy examples from practice that will allow you to practise and develop your skills, thus encouraging problem-solving approaches relating to nursing practice. It is suggested that you keep a numeracy journal as you work your way through this book. The advice is to keep your reflections short and to the point to allow the focus to be on actually practising your numeracy skills as they relate to practice. All chapters will conclude with advice to reflect on learning and develop action plans to ensure that you continue to practise numeracy skills learned.

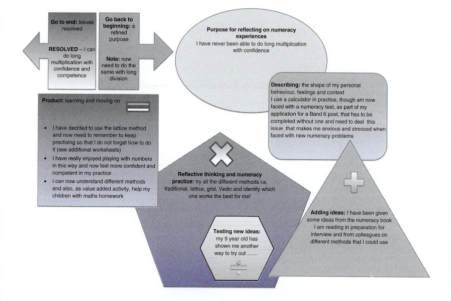

The language of the book

The primary target audience of this book is nurses who work with children and young people or students who are planning to become nurses, although clearly not all readers will be nurses so, in this case, please forgive the focus and use of the word 'nurse' throughout. All the content is relevant and useful to other healthcare professionals, even though it is set within the context of nursing policy related to skills and competences. The Standards for Pre-registration Nursing Education and Essential Skills Clusters (2010) form the guiding framework for numeracy skills acquisition for this book, although opportunities to explore the world of numeracy/mathematics are also taken so as to offer different dimensions on this world, thus generating interest and new perspectives.

References and bibliography

The references used within each chapter will appear at the end of the book, along with a bibliography, useful websites and other resources.

Glossary of terms

Numeracy terms will be defined within the related chapters.

Do you need a calculator as part of your numeracy toolkit?

Many nurses are totally dependent on calculators when completing numeracy assessments and calculations in practice, whether at pre-registration or post-registration level, and there is allowance to do so. The NMC line is as follows:

> The use of calculators to determine the volume or quantity of medication should not act as a substitute for arithmetical knowledge and skill.

> (NMC, 2007, updated 2012)

From this statement there is a clear message that all nurses should be able to do numeracy-related activity in relation to administration of drugs at the very least without the use of a calculator. This book aims to help nurses achieve this and use a calculator as a back-up and second checker rather than as a first-line approach. The advice then is that the calculator is part of your toolkit as a back-up to check answers! As a result, if you happen not to have easy access to a calculator, you will still be able to numerate.

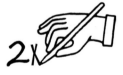

Diagnostic self-assessment

Start by having a go at the diagnostic assessment (Answers at the back of the book). This will allow you to identify your level of numeracy competency as a benchmark and where you may need to focus your attention, especially if revising or preparing for a numeracy assessment or test.

SECTION 1: Numbers and place value

Write the following numbers in full (in words for 1–4 and numbers in 5–8)

1. 652
2. 5,989
3. 12,564
4. 167,700
5. Sixty-seven and three-hundredths
6. Three hundred and seventy-five and a half
7. Seventy thousand, nine hundred and ninety-nine
8. Seven million, five thousand and forty-seven
9. Define: What is an ordinal number?
10. Write down the first seven prime numbers in order from smallest to largest.

SECTION 2: Weights and measures

1. Sally, a student nurse, drinks 375 mL out of half litre carton of juice – how much is left?
2. Convert 4.65 grams to milligrams.
3. What is the combined weight of two store crates delivered to the ward weighing 2.3 kg, and 3¼ kg and two packets weighing 750 grams and 0.5 kg?
4. You have a 3 litre jug that is full of water. How many 175 mL glasses of water can you pour out of this jug and what is the remainder?

5. Sarah's temperature rises from 38.5°C to 39.6°C – by how much has it risen?
6. Simon weighs 49 kg when weighed fully clothed on the ward scales. His clothes weigh 1.7 kg. What is his weight unclothed?
7. It takes 13 minutes to walk to children's outpatients. You need to be there by 2.45 PM – what time do you set off to get there just in time using the 24 hour clock?

Here is a list of departments that you regularly go to from Gamma Ward with children and their parents at Arch Mede Hospital.

A & E:	**245 metres**
Children's Outpatient Department:	**275 metres**
ENT Clinic:	**259 metres**
Pharmacy:	**280 metres**
Plaster Room:	**232 metres**
X-Ray Department:	**195 metres**

8. Which department is closest to Gamma Ward?
9. You go backwards and forwards to pharmacy three times – how far have you walked?
10. Which department is furthest away from Gamma Ward?

SECTION 3: Basic numeracy skills, i.e. addition, subtraction, long multiplication and long division

Add together the following numbers

1. 76 and 38 =
2. 4.78 + 5.84 =

Subtract the following numbers

3. 365 from 1087 =
4. 16.66 – 7.87 =
5. Multiply 34 by 6
6. 479 × 9 =

7. Calculate the product of 18 and 13
8. Divide 360 by 12
9. What are the factors of 36?
10. 133 chocolates are shared equally among 14 staff on a children's ward. How many sweets does each nurse receive and what is the remainder?

SECTION 4: Fractions, percentages, ratio and proportion

1. Reduce 95/120 to its lowest terms?
2. Convert 75/20 into a mixed number fraction
3. Define what is a vulgar fraction
4. 7¼ – 3¾ =
5. Multiply ½ by ¼
6. Convert 4/16 into a percentage
7. Write down 17/20 as a decimal number
8. What is 30% of 950?
9. You have been asked to dilute some juice 1 part to 4 of water to make up a glass equalling 200 mL. How much water do you add?
10. How much glucose is there in a 500 mL bag of 5% dextrose?

SECTION 5: Using formulae in children's nursing practice

1. How much should a 6-month-old baby weigh approximately?
2. Paracetamol has been prescribed at a dose of 15 mg/kg for a 6-year-old child who has pain following grommet insertion. He weighs 19 kg. How much will be prescribed?
3. It is supplied in a liquid formulation 250 mg in 5 mL. How much will be administered?
4. An infant is prescribed 600 micrograms of a drug that is available in a liquid form of 1 mg in 2 mL. What amount will be given to the infant?
5. An antibiotic has been prescribed to a 4-year-old boy post appendicectomy, it is available as 500 mg in 100 mL bag and he has been prescribed 160 mg

to be administered intravenously. How much will be given?

6. It was given at 13.30 and is prescribed 8 hourly – what time is the next dose due?

7. Calculate the Body Mass Index for a child who weighs 20 kg and is 115 cm tall rounded to one decimal place.

8. Calculate the body surface area for a child who weighs 12.5 kg and is 88 cm tall and round to two decimal places.

9. You are reconstituting a drug in a vial following these instructions: You need to add 1.2 mL of diluent to make up a solution of 75 mg in 2 mL. What is the displacement value?

10. The prescribed dose is 15 mg – how much will you give?

How well have you performed?

Identify the areas where you have made errors and record as part of your personal development planning. This will then give you some idea of the sections within the book that you need to concentrate on. There are further practice assessments throughout the book so that you can monitor your progress. Even when you have completed the activities in the book there are more worksheets on the website (ONE) to allow you to return and practise further. As you can see, mathematical language needs to be understood in order to be able to do the calculation itself and it is this that quite often confuses nurses in terms of understanding how the problem is defined.

Recording your achievements

Clearly the fact that you have more confidence in your numeracy competency is the main reward for working your way through this book, although once you have completed the book to the extent identified in your personal development plan, please feel free to print off a certificate which appears on ONE to add to your professional portfolio. We nurse children and young people and there is no better reward than stickers, gold stars and certificates both for children and adults alike!

Answers

SECTION		ANSWER	HOW DID YOU DO?	ADVICE
Section 1: Place Value and Number	1	Six hundred and fifty-two		Chapter 1 focuses in the basics of numerical notation taking you back to what you learned when you were at primary school and which most people forget because they did learn this when they were little. This Chapter will reintroduce you to the exciting world of numbers!
	2	Five thousand nine hundred and eighty-nine		
	3	Twelve thousand five hundred and sixty-four		
	4	One hundred and sixty seven thousand and seven hundred		
	5	67.05		
	6	375.5		
	7	70,999		
	8	7,005,047		
	9	The order of numbers in a set i.e. first, second etc.		
	10	2,3,5,7,11,13,17		
Section 2: Weights and Measures	1	125 mL		Chapter 2 covers the use of measures in children's nursing practice and will explore all aspects of use of counting and SI units. Have you used the correct units, written correctly throughout?
	2	4650 mg		
	3	6.8 kg		
	4	17/25 mL		
	5	1.1°C		
	6	47.3 kg		
	7	14.32 hrs		
	8	X-Ray		
	9	1.682 km		
	10	Pharmacy		

SECTION		ANSWER	HOW DID YOU DO?	ADVICE
Section 3: Basic Numeracy Skills	1	114		Chapter 3 covers a back to basic approach for doing addition, subtraction, division and multiplication for you to be able to learn different ways of performing these operations without a calculator.
	2	10.62		
	3	722		
	4	8.79		
	5	204		
	6	4311		
	7	234		
	8	30		
	9	1, 2, 3, 4, 6, 9, 12, 18 and 36		
	10	9.5 or 9 with 7 remaining		
Section 4: Ratio, Proportion and Percentages	1	19/24		Chapter 4 explores the world of parts of the whole in the form of fractions, percentages, ratio and proportion as it applies to the children's nursing world.
	2	3¾		
	3	A fraction with number above a line and a number below the line – a common fraction!		
	4	3½		
	5	1/8		
	6	25%		
	7	85%		
	8	285		
	9	160 mL		
	10	25 g		

SECTION		ANSWER	HOW DID YOU DO?	ADVICE
Section 5: Using Nursing Formulae	1	7 kg		Chapter 5 puts all the pieces together to explore the use of equations and formulae in children's nursing practice as well as the administration of medication to children and young people. Chapter 6 focuses on more complex calculations as applied to the very young and vulnerable i.e. the neonate. This will enable you to start thinking about more specialist children's nursing practice and the complexity that may apply to use of number also as well to as to explore more complex use of number just out of interest.
	2	285 mg		
	3	5.7 mL		
	4	1.2 mL		
	5	32 mL		
	6	21:30 hrs		
	7	15.1		
	8	0.55 m²		
	9	0.8 mL		
	10	0.4 mL		
TOTAL (out of 50)				

Chapter 1

· ·

THE ROLE OF NUMERACY IN NURSING AND HEALTHCARE PRACTICE

Numeracy in Children's Nursing, First Edition. Arija Parker
© 2015 John Wiley & Sons, Ltd. Published 2015 by John Wiley & Sons Ltd.

LEARNING FOCUS

The Role of Numeracy in Nursing

The broad focus of this chapter is to define what numeracy is and where numeracy skills are needed in healthcare settings. There will be a particular focus on nursing practice and, more specifically, on numeracy skills to support children and young people's nursing.

LEARNING OUTCOMES

By the end of this chapter you should be able to:

- Identify why you need to read this book and why it is important to your practice
- Define what numeracy/mathematics are
- Have a conceptual understanding of the problems that adults, and so by default nurses have in relation to the use of number
- Use place value and the denary system
- Reflect on what you would like to achieve by working through this book and companion website having completed the diagnostic assessment which precedes this chapter

CASE SCENARIO 1

Una Venn (Age 4) is visiting the hospital for a preoperative visit and assessment prior to admission for day case surgery in the following week for ENT surgery (tonsillectomy, adenoidectomy and insertion of grommets). She is accompanied by her mother, Mrs. Venn and little brother, Jack (1 year).

Una gets to visit ENT theatre 1 together with other children who will be coming into hospital for various day case surgical procedures over the coming week. Both Mrs. Venn and Una have the documentation explained to them, including a Pain Assessment Chart. The nurse, who will be caring for Una, carries out a set of baseline observations and weighs Una and then gives them both a chance to ask questions. Mrs. Venn is also advised about pain management in hospital, postoperatively and on discharge. The nursing staff on Gamma Ward use the Arch Mede Hospital Pain Assessment Tool for children. (The Arch Mede Pain assessment too is a fictitious tool just for use to illustrate numeracy issues in this book. It is adapted from Baker and Wong (1983; 1988) and numerous other numerical, visual and colour analogue scales and has a number focused theme.)

She had some blood tests, including a full blood count (FBC), performed in clinic the week before and the results are included in the table below. Mum is informed of the result and reassured that all is fine in preparation for admission to hospital and theatre next week.

Una had a FBC performed because she has been unwell recently and looked pale and anaemic when seen by the ENT doctor in clinic. A FBC is not routinely performed as part of a preoperative assessment.

Hospital number	AMH2014-01
Ward name/number	Gamma Ward 3 (children's day case surgical unit)

Temperature	Pulse	Blood pressure	Respirations	CRT	Pain score	PEWS score
37°C	106 bpm	Not recorded	26 per minute	1–2 seconds	0	0

Full blood count	Una's result	Normal range
Haemoglobin	13.3 g/dL	13.8 g/dL
White cell count	7×10^9/L	$4–12 \times 10^9$/L
Platelets	255×10^9/L	$100–300 \times 10^9$/L

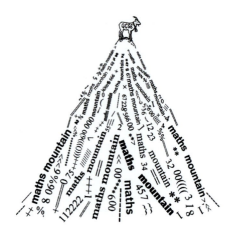

INTRODUCTION

This chapter will explore the context of numeracy practice in nursing in general and children and young people's nursing more specifically, define what is numeracy/mathematics and introduce the beginnings and basics of numeracy language including place value and the use of zero.

Why read this book?

The first question to ask is why are you reading this book and why do we need yet another book on numeracy for healthcare, nursing and children's nursing in particular, especially when there are already many other very good numeracy text books available.

You only need to look at the unfortunately regular news headlines lambasting nurses for their poor numerical abilities, which lead to serious prescription and drug administration errors. As a result we need to sit up and take note of the fact that we need to be constantly updating and developing our numeracy skills however numeracy competent we may feel we are. Whilst competence is needed for all fields of nursing, with the nursing of children and young people – where we care for neonates to adolescent patients – being accurate, safe and competent in numeracy practice is of vital importance. In addition, the numeracy subset of skills for this particular group of patients also serves to offer more challenges to numerical ability.

So, to delve a bit more deeply beyond media headlines alone to more research-based evidence, the National Patient Safety Agency (2007a) found that the most serious errors were caused by errors in medicine administration (41%) and prescribing (32%). Medication errors with children were reported from all stages of the medication process though the majority were from the part involving administration of the medicine itself (56%). The main causes are listed below:

- **Prescribing errors** – where medicines prescribed as volume of liquid rather than actual dose and also calculation errors, that is, 5 mL instead of 250 mg
- **Dispensing errors** – due to labelling errors
- **Administration** – involving, most commonly, intravenous drug errors though also giving a drug like paracetamol when previous dose given was not recorded, a drug being given to the wrong patient or giving the wrong amount, that is, millilitre instead of milligram

Additionally, there is a whole list of errors including wrong dose, strength or frequency errors, weighing scale errors and weight in pounds not kilograms. This is why this book has a focus on **all** aspects of numeracy, not just that related to medication administration. The most common medicines involved are paracetamol, gentamicin and morphine, which are all medicines that are commonly given to children and young people and are used as examples in Chapter 6, when focusing in on the needs of our neonatal patients. Here is the justification for reading and learning from a book that has a focus on the whole range of basic numeracy skills with a focus on the particular needs of children and young people.

So why do nurses who care for children make numerical mistakes? Whilst a lack of understanding of the basics could be one reason for the poor numeracy skills of nursing students, registered children's nurses and the nursing population in general, there are other issues that might explain why there is a deficit in these skills. There is a commonly held perception, that is common in British people, not only nurses, of 'I can't do maths', which may be a cultural factor though could also be due to lack of confidence, dyscalculia and maths anxiety. This is well reported in the literature including Pozehl (1996) who found that nursing students demonstrated higher levels of maths anxiety than other students. Whilst, anecdotally, it would appear that we do not have nurses who have dyscalculia working in clinical areas, probably because of a Grade C pass in maths GSCE as an entry gate to programmes of nurse training, there are many prospective nursing students who spend many years attempting to meet this entry gate to the profession by repeating courses and redoing the examinations until they pass and meet the entry criteria. Whilst they have the 'certificate' this does not mean that they have confidence in their numerical ability. They then spend the next 3 years of the course and beyond worrying about every numeracy test and assessment that comes their way. Increasingly now students have to pass a numeracy assessment as part of the recruitment process both to get entry onto a nursing programme and then to gain employment on registration. From a professional perspective there are also the ethical and moral issues to think about if you are practising without numerical proficiency.

It could also be argued that even the most proficient nurse mathematician still has these feelings of anxiety when faced with tests, so for all who are reading and utilising this book to improve their numeracy skills, the message of 'practice, practice, practice' will form the basis of advice offered. Whilst the message so far has been very serious, it is really important to emphasise that having some fun with numbers is the best way to learn, which is the approach this book would like to take by also looking at how children learn about numbers.

How do we know if we are numerate?

Numeracy is 'of or relating to numbers', where to be numerate 'is the ability to use numbers especially in arithmetical operations'. The ability to be numerate is clearly linked to literacy which is the 'ability to read and write and the ability to use language proficiently' (Collins

English Dictionary, 1999). This is reflected in the famous quotation as below:

> [The universe] cannot be read until we have learnt the language and become familiar with the characters in which it is written. It is written in mathematical language, and the letters are triangles, circles and other geometrical figures, without which means it is humanly impossible to comprehend a single word.
>
> (Galileo Galilei, *Opere II Saggiatore*, p. 171)

Goldbeck (1999) (cited in Rothman et al., 2008) states that numeracy consists of four main skills:

1. Basic – identifying numbers
2. Computational – simple manipulation of numbers
3. Analytical – inference, estimation, proportions
4. Statistical

Rothman et al. (2008) basically define numeracy as the ability to understand and use numbers in daily life, so we could conclude by stating that numeracy for nurses is all about the ability to identify, compute, analyse numbers that relate to nursing practice and utilise them effectively to ensure safe practice.

The fact that literacy and numeracy walk together hand in hand cannot be overemphasised where you have probably already realised that how a nursing numeracy question is written and phrased has a major impact on your comprehension. It can often be difficult to actually unpick the written language with respect to what have you been asked to do. Once this is done the numeracy problem is usually easy to solve.

The teaching of numeracy skills in pre- and post-registration nursing curricula

So if we acknowledge that we have a need for further numeracy education for nurses why are we not doing anything about it? How are we teaching numeracy skills in practice and in education settings? Why are we, as professional nurses, not acknowledging that there are deficits in knowledge via reflective practice and doing something about it?

From a brief overview of the research into nursing ability or disability as may be the case, Goldin (1990) found that overemphasis on the use of formulae in nurse education is potentially damaging to students because it involves rote learning what they may perceive to be meaningless information. This is reflected in the way children learn and are taught mathematics (see Chapter 7). Baroody and Ginsburg (1990) go on to say that systematic calculation errors or 'bugs' learnt in this way ensure that student cannot see any sense in what they do and blindly accept the results of what they do. Gillies (2004) emphasises the importance of learning mathematics with understanding so that processes, when performing drug calculations, are understood, more easily remembered and more easily transferred to other situations.

Do you recognise any of these characteristics in yourself?

Needless to say, there is a much greater emphasis on numeracy in nursing curricula and moving beyond rote learning practices to teach about number in Higher Education settings though the degree to which we should teach these skills is debatable and too big a topic area for this little book.

From this introductory discussion it is clear that we need to start at the beginning in developing and building on our existing numeracy knowledge and so need to introduce the concept of 'place value' into this chapter. This will then correct any initial misconceptions that there may be about numbers including:

- conceptions of how numbers behave (particularly in relation to fractions which is an area that is frequently highlighted as that of worry and anxiety from work with pre-registration nursing students – see Chapter 4),
- trying to ensure that the vocabulary used is clear in terms of how we use language – literacy and

oracy, including nursing jargon, as well as the use of mathematics language,

- focusing in on correct procedures and methods, which will then help problem solving with respect to choosing the correct operation to use. This should then stop the frequent behaviour of guessing that students may use as a strategy, especially when being tested using multiple choice questions.

This does not mean that we stop using the classic nursing rule/formula, that many of us have learned, which works well for many nurses. We need to ensure that all appreciate and understand the numeracy/mathematics that underpins the formula – in this case the children's nursing formula. In fact we look at this in much greater detail in Chapter 5.

From a numeracy perspective the following quotation is the Gold Standard in relation to nursing with numbers in this book and is as follows:

> To be numerate means to be competent, confident and comfortable with one's own judgements on how to use mathematics in a particular situation and if so what mathematics to use, how to do it, what degree of accuracy is appropriate and what the answer means in relation to the context.
>
> (Coben, 2000, p.35)

This is included as part of the NMC Standards for Pre-registration Nurse Education – Annexe 3 Essential Skills Clusters (2010) adapted and written as 'The focus should be on demonstration of competence and confidence with regard to judgements on whether to use calculations in a particular situation and, if so, what calculations to use, how to do it, what degree of accuracy is appropriate, and what the answer means in relation to the context'.

This statement is the pillar of this book with respect to looking at the three numeracy (or calculation) C's of competence, confidence and comfort!

'Calculate competently, confidently and comfortably' could be the motto for this book!

Clarifying our understanding of what dyscalculia is

Whilst most nurses who have a perception that they are not good at mathematics have a problem with competence, confidence and/or comfort, there are a group of adults, including nurses, whose problems with numbers are more complex. Dyscalculia is a 'condition that affects the ability to acquire arithmetical skills, where those affected have difficulty understanding simple number concepts, lack an intuitive grasp of numbers and have problems learning facts' (Dfes, 2001). The Royal College of Nursing has explored the issue of dyslexia, dyscalculia and dyspraxia amongst the nursing population to identify the scale of the 'problem' so as to develop a strategy for how to deal with the needs these nurses have. Anecdotally, from many years of experience in nursing practice and contradicting the statement made in the previous paragraph, there is no doubt that there are registered nurses with dyscalculia in practice! The following materials will help you develop some insight into the problems some people have with numeracy and the strategies they develop to manage their dyscalculia. The focus of this book goes beyond just improving your own skills to also thinking about how to assess numerical ability in others and gain more understanding in how to teach numeracy skills within a nursing context to children and their parents/carers who may also struggle with numbers and how to use them.

Access the following online resources to find out more.

Dyslexia, dyspraxia and dyscalculia – guide for managers and practitioners (RCN, 2010)
http://www.rcn.org.uk/__data/assets/pdf_file/0006/333537/003833.pdf

Dyslexia, dyspraxia and dyscalculia – toolkit for nursing staff (RCN, 2010)
http://www.rcn.org.uk/__data/assets/pdf_file/0003/333534/003835.pdf

Dyslexia, dyspraxia and dyscalculia – a pocket guide (RCN, 2011)
http://www.rcn.org.uk/__data/assets/pdf_file/0007/372994/003851.pdf

Learning theories and social context

Whilst it seems obvious to say that a context is essential to the learning of skills such as numeracy why is this so? Hansman (2001) argues that social context is central to learning, particularly to learning in adulthood. She goes on to explore issues around social learning theories focusing in on the fact that the setting provides the tools and mechanisms that aid and structure the learning process and the social setting itself provides a learning context that determines the learning that takes place. Clearly it is vital, for a nurse learning numeracy skills, to do so within a nursing setting and context, within a framework of nursing skills and competences, using nursing tools and theory, thus enhancing the numeracy learning experience for children's nurses. This book aims to set all the numeracy activities within a children's nursing context to aid the learning process. This is the reason why case scenarios are included in all the chapters of this book. We could add 'Context' to our calculation motto.

This book does not stand alone in numeracy for nursing learning and teaching. As already demonstrated, this book will make reference to other numeracy-related texts. There is a rich tapestry of books and resources that already exist and thus enhances this text book and resources also. We cannot use a 'one size fits all approach'.

THE LANGUAGE OF MATHEMATICS AND NUMERACY

Mathematics versus numeracy – the same or different?

For the purposes of this book, as reflected in the title, the word numeracy will be used as the core term to define common understanding, though, in theory, there is no difference between the words mathematics or numeracy as used and they can be used interchangeably. The word mathematics will appear here and there because it could be argued that it is the more commonly recognised word.

The Collins English Dictionary (1999) defines mathematics as 'a group of sciences including algebra, geometry and calculus concerned with the study of number, quantity, shape and space and their interrelationship by using a specialised notation' and numeracy as 'of or relating to numbers' which does appear to suggest that numeracy is something less scientific or rigorous than what mathematics is, that is, mathematics is a science and numeracy has a more practical perspective. What do you think?

It is worth reflecting on your definition of the words mathematics and numeracy at this point:

- Use the PDP template to explore what the words mean to you – are they different or the same? Does this matter?
- Which word will you use when discussing number-related activity with children in clinical practice?

Introducing numerical concepts and ideas

Five important areas of numeracy language will be covered in this section – that is defining numbers, place value, number bases, the value of zero and prime numbers.

1. What are numbers?

What follows is a definition of 'number'

- An arithmetical value, expressed by a word, symbol or figure, representing a particular quantity and used in counting and making calculations and for showing order in a series or for identification.

This can then be subdivided down into defining a numeral and then cardinal, ordinal and nominal numbers.

- A **numeral** is a symbol for the idea of what we call a number.
- A **cardinal number** is how many there are of a thing and can also be called counting numbers because they define quantity.

- **Ordinal numbers** tell the order of things in a set – first, second, third, etc. Ordinal numbers do not show quantity. They only show rank or position, that is, like the chapters in this book which place skills learned in a certain order.
- A **nominal number** names something – a telephone number, a player on a team. Nominal numbers do not show quantity or rank. They are used only to identify something such as Una and her hospital number.

We give a number a symbol though it also has a word associated with it. The English language does not help in relation to how syllables are used to construct words which reflect a numerical value. For example there are three forms in relation to 'three' as a unit, which as a unit of ten becomes 'thirteen' though with the addition of twenty becomes 'thirty'. Only as a unit in hundreds does the relationship become clear, that is, three hundred. Where is the sense here when trying to understand how to count numbers? (Sousa, 2008)

Interestingly, it has been found that Asian children learn to count earlier than Western children partly due to the simplicity of their number syntax, which again reflects the close relationship between literacy and numeracy.

2. Everything in its place and a place for everything

Place value is all about number representation systems and the meaning applied to numbers, which within the denary system that we use here involves the use of number in relation to 100s, 10s and units (of one). Sharma (1993) states that not only do students (children in his situation and context) need to understand the value of digits/numbers they also need to have spatial awareness in terms of orientation and space organisation. This is where problems arise in adult learners as well as children. According to Sharma (1993) place value is the language of mathematics – 'a true symbol system'. He sees the development of place value system as a 'truly great achievement of human ingenuity'. He goes on to state that place value is a demonstration of the key characteristics of maths thinking: efficiency, elegance and exactness, which clearly underpins learner understanding and progression in their numeracy learning. Place value forms the basis of all that follows number wise in numeracy education, so without a command and understanding of why we need to value 'place' people will struggle with numeracy. This is clearly demonstrated in numeracy teaching practice where errors in 'exactness' mean that numbers get mixed up and you end up with an incorrect answer.

MILLIONS	HUNDRED THOUSANDS	TEN THOUSANDS	THOUSANDS	HUNDREDS	TENS	UNITS	DECIMAL POINT	TENTHS	HUNDREDTHS	THOUSANDTHS
1 000 000	100 000	10 000	1000	100	10	1	.	0.1	0.01	0.001
8	6	5	4	3	2	1	.	1	2	3
							.			
							.			
							.			
							.			
							.			
							.			
							.			
							.			
							.			
							.			

Definition of place value.

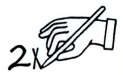

Practice adding the following numbers to the chart above or on the online version. Also write in your own numbers and then say them aloud!

- Sixty-five and three-tenths
- Seven thousand and seventy-seven
- Eight million, nine hundred and eighty-five thousand, five hundred and twenty-two

To sum up this section on place value Sharma (1993) does argue that 'mastery' of the place value system is an important milestone for children and if this is not understood they cannot proceed to understand other mathematical concepts and principles. This has not been mastered by many nurses so it is worth spending time ensuring that you understand place value so please complete some of the activities before moving on.

Using graph or squared paper allows you to offer due respect to the place value of a number and will reduce the chance of making mistakes! See Section 3 on ONE to print off some squared graph paper.

Within nursing practice we tend to proceed to more complex numerical problems (by using a formula), where multiple steps with regard to manipulation of numbers need to be taken, using a problem-solving approach, without checking out whether we understand the meaning of place value.

When working with really big numbers it is useful to use the exponential form by use of the 'power' of a number. You will encounter this way of writing large numbers when looking at blood results. So for example $10 \times 10 \times 10 \times 10$ = 10,000 (ten thousand) though this could be written 10^4.

So if we look at Una's FBC result you can see that both white cell and platelet counts are recorded in units of $\times 10^9$/L, which makes the numbers much more manageable, even though they are unbelievably big numbers.

3. Number bases

The denary system is the number base that we use to work with numbers, that is, base 10. The denary (or decimal) numbering system is the most widely used in the world. It has a base of 10 and uses the numerals 0, 1, 2, 3, 4, 5, 6, 7, 8, 9. Working in tens is much easier than any number which explains why this system is so widely used. We use the denary system in nursing practice and calculations, which should become apparent when we look at other bases that could be used.

In nursing practice it would be uncommon to explore other number bases, though it is worth introducing this idea of base into this chapter for the very fact that it is an interesting topic area, which also offers us a greater understanding of what place value actually means. The historical context is particularly meaningful when we used pounds, shilling and pence as used prior to 1970, pre-decimalisation, and in very complex calculations when calculating insulin dosages, which did not always follow the metric system in terms of the now accepted standard 100 units per millilitre formulation that we use now. This can still be remembered by many nurses. The pre-decimal system did not use a standardised system of units in relation to different formulations of insulin and this caused great confusion to healthcare professionals and patients' alike, that is, with differing amounts in different volumes depending on the type of insulin used, which meant that nurses had to work in a different base system for each calculation.[1]

Interestingly, the old USP unit of insulin was arbitrarily set to the amount required to reduce the concentration of blood glucose in a fasting rabbit to 45 mg/dL[2]. It is clear that the decision to rationalise the situation in the 1970s was a very wise move to reduce prescribing errors made by medical staff and administration errors made by nurses and patients themselves. To add some confusion to the present situation though, in some veterinary care setting and in other countries the usage of a 40 unit/mL concentration of insulin is common (Hanas, 2010). This has an impact when giving advice to children and

---

[1]That is not to say that the present system is easy to use and understand. The present system of 100 units per millilitre can still be confusing because of the small volumes of insulin administered (in relation to small children particularly) and the different sizes of insulin syringe that are available, that is, 0.3, 0.5 and 1 mL, though it has to be noted that most children are now using pens to administer insulin thus avoiding confusion with syringe choice. Even now the situation is not straightforward because international units do not follow the usual convention of SI units, that is, one international unit of insulin is the biological equivalent of 45.5 micrograms of pure crystalline insulin. Administration of insulin will be discussed further in Chapter 7.

[2]A decilitre is equal to 100 mL or one-tenth of a litre.

families when travelling overseas should their supplies of U-100 insulin run out or expire. This advice will be offered by nurses who need to give advice based on assessment of numeracy ability of their clients (child and family) as well as have the skills to ensure accurate conversions and safe practice.

This could then lead us on to explore other bases out of interest, that is, binary systems (which are used routinely in the computing world) and we will look at base 6 in relation to time in the next chapter. It is also interesting to explore other number systems such as the use of Roman numerals which are used frequently when teaching subjects like anatomy and physiology, that is, naming of cranial nerves and whilst we have no need to learn how to add, subtract, multiply and divide using different number bases, some examples are offered on ONE for you to practice and play with if this topic area interests and fascinates you. Also of interest is that the Romans did not develop the idea of place value at all from what had gone before historically in the development of mathematical knowledge – it was already in existence in other countries. This allows us to explore numeral systems in terms of whether they are positional and how they use zero, which leads us on to another important discussion around zero as a 'place holder'.

From observation it is clear that children's nurses use their fingers a lot to count so we have to think about the Roman system again. The word 'digit' as used for numbers comes from the Latin word for finger and numeral and Roman numerals originally represented fingers.

The greatest brain activity is in the left parietal lobe and also in the region of the motor cortex that controls the fingers – is this a coincidence? (Dehaene et al., 2004)

4. The value of zero

You have probably not thought about it before but why is the digit zero so important?

Connor and Robertson (2000) state what is commonly held in that there are two uses of zero which are very important though very different. One use is as an empty place indicator in our place value number system, as already discussed, so that in a number like 5505 the zero is used so that the positions of the 5 and 500 are correct. If we miss out the zero the number is completely different, that is, 555. The second use of zero is as a number in itself. Connor and Robertson (2000) talk about the history of zero and about the differing aspects of zero – the concept, the notation and the name where the name comes from the Arabic 'sifr' meaning 'cipher'.

Access ONE to find out more if you are interested!

As you will have gathered this is a difficult concept to understand particularly when we think of the value of zero as 'nought' or 'nothing'. When it is a label on a graph you can clearly see it does have value though if you want to quantify it as an object in your hand then clearly there is nothing there. No other numbers have more than one name which either identifies it as something special or something that is different maybe.

With respect to our work with zeros, they are extremely valuable as a position holder (see Chapter 3 when working with long division), though sometimes are not helpful, that is, when they appear after a decimal point and do not hold the position of numbers after a decimal point, that is, 5.05 the zero is needed. When looking at 5.50 the zero is not needed – it is five point five (or five and five-tenths) not five point fifty (which is an error that many children make when talking about numbers not realising that they should be thinking about fifty-hundredths which is the same as five-tenths). So if you have a drug prescribed as 100 mg do not be tempted to add a decimal point and lots of trailing zeroes at the end, that is, 100.00 mg – you can immediately see why errors could occur! Trailing zeroes have been identified as a potential source of serious drug errors (DH, 2004).

5. Prime numbers

A prime number can only be divided by 1 and the number itself with no remainder. Why is this important to know and why are these numbers so interesting?

Enzensberger (2006) calls prime numbers prima donna[3] numbers which is a great way of describing numbers that do stand out as being different. Why do we need to appreciate this difference and how does it help us appreciate and solve nursing-related number problems?

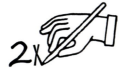

Here are some prime numbers with some of them missing – can you identify the missing numbers?

2		5	7		13
17	19		29	31	
41	43	47		59	61
	71	73	79	83	
	101		107		113

Also answer the question: Why does 1 not count?

Why is it useful to know your prime numbers?

This helps you understand when you can cancel down and simplify particularly fractions where speed is of the essence, that is, in timed numeracy tests and in some emergency situations. Prime numbers cannot be made any simpler which is why they behave like prima donnas.

Numbers and patterns

The Fibonacci series (created by Leonardo Fibonacci in 1202) is a series of numbers that famously originated

---

[3]A prima donna is literally translated as 'first lady'. The term is used to describe the female lead in an opera or opera company and can also be used when describing a very temperamental person with an inflated view of their own talent or importance (OED). A diva could be another term for prima donna though this term is usually applied to a lady who is talented though knows that she is temperamental or haughty. A prime number could be a prima donna and a diva.

around the mating patterns of rabbits where you start with 1 + 1 and then chart how they multiply which generates the number sequence. The first two numbers in the series are one and one. To obtain each number of the series, you simply add the two numbers that came before it. In other words, each number of the series is the sum of the two numbers preceding it. 1 + 1 = 2; 2 + 1 = 3; 3 + 2 = 5; 5 + 3 = 8 and so on to infinity. Fibonacci (and those who have come after him to study this branch of mathematics) then found that this identifies patterns in nature, that is, shells (the Fibonacci spiral) and flowers (with the arrangement of petals) and the way trees grow from one trunk to branches. The tree illustration in Chapter 7 will also form the same principles in the way it grows from a single trunk, to branches and sub-branches.

This demonstrates why numeracy is so interesting and how it applies to the world around us. Children also find this fascinating so it is a good discussion point as well as play activity in generating the series. The numbers and patterns create a good play and distraction activity whereby generating the series is good fun for children. The pattern starts with 1, 1, 2, 3, 5, 8, 13, 21 and then carries on to infinity.[4]

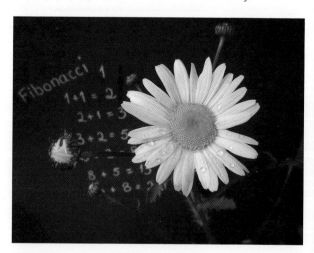

A Daisy's petals show the Fibonacci pattern.

---

[4] Infinity is a number greater than any assignable quantity or countable number (symbol = ∞).

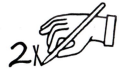

When looking at Una's medical notes, what are the issues that may arise when using her hospital number?

From this brief introduction to numbers and, in conclusion, we will return to nurses and numeracy practice by identifying some of the common errors that occur when working with numbers.

ERRORS IN NUMERACY PRACTICE

Identified in the table below are some common reasons for errors and misconceptions in numeracy. Can you relate to any of these? In addition to completing the pretest it is worth identifying some of the common errors you make as part of your personal and professional development activity that could form part of your journey through this book.

Error	Reason and examples
Conceptual error	Not understanding the concept e.g ½ is one whole one divided into two equal parts
Vocabulary	Unfamiliar vocabulary (product, divisibility, factor, etc.), misunderstood vocabulary, which applies if your first language is not English and also when you first learned to 'do' maths
Wrong operation	Chooses the wrong operation
Defective procedure/ method	Errors in carrying out the steps in a correctly chosen operation
Overgeneralisation	Rules learned, then applied where they do not work i.e. × 100 means add 2 zeros, so 1.3 × 100 must be 1.300
Undergeneralisation	E.g. 'since 5 × 7 = 7 × 5, then 24 ÷ 4 must equal 4 ÷ 24', or '8 + 2 = 2 + 8, so 8 − 2 must be equal to 2 − 8'
Random response	A guess!

So what are the common errors and misconceptions that occur with nurses and adults in general and why do they occur? Some observations made include the way a nurse may actually write down numbers and sums with total nonregard for place value, using tiny numbers, in the corner of a page that also is usually full of other information. This appears to be done in a secretive way as if they do not want others to see what they are doing, that is, like children who cover up their work so others cannot see what they are doing. Many of us try to hide away when wanting to be able to concentrate on working something out which in the context of needing peace and quiet to calculate medication dosages is a good thing though we need to be open about how we are doing the calculations and share good practice.

The following may seem overly simplistic; though it is a very effective advice, that is, write numbers clearly in large letters/numbers on a blank piece of paper with a clear respect for place value – see ONE for downloadable square/graph paper.

APPLICATION OF NUMBER TO CASE SCENARIO

And finally, to return to Una and her family whilst visiting the ward on a preoperative assessment. In relation to the use of number we will focus on her observations and the use and explanation of a pain assessment tool.

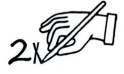

- The normal ranges of observations for different ages appear in ONE and in the next Chapter 2 – do Una's baseline observations fit within the normal range?
- How would you explain what the smiley faces mean to a 4-year-old child, like Una and would you expect her to understand the numerical meanings attached to the chart as it appears below, which consists of a visual scale, a numerical scale, a colour scale (on ONE) and a pain descriptor scale?

The conclusive answer to this question appears in Chapter 7 where the focus is on looking at how children make meaning of and from number though what follows is some explanation.

0	1	2	3	4
No pain	A little bit of pain	More than a little pain	Lots of pain	The worst pain

Arch Mede Faces Pain Scale.

Source: Adapted into the Arch Mede Hospital Children's Shape Pain Assessment tool from multiple sources including Wong–Baker FACES™ Pain Rating Scale (1983)

Note: Replace the word 'pain' with the words for pain used by the child and family.

 See ONE Section 1 for a colour version of pain scale incorporating a colour analogue scale.

Assessing pain in children and young people

Una will be in pain following surgery so it is really important to help prepare both Una and her mum for what is going to happen when she comes into hospital which includes an explanation of the pain assessment chart used on Gamma Ward. This includes a numerical element which will also be discussed in the next chapter.

 Refer to the RCN (2009) Recognition and Assessment of Acute Pain in Children for more information about pain management.
http://www.rcn.org.uk/development/practice/clinicalguidelines/pain

Which pain assessment tool for which age group?

The suggestion is that we use different tools for different ages as follows:

- 0–3 years observer scores (with parent or nurse recording the pain score)

- 3–8 years faces pain scale
- >8 years faces/numerical scales

It makes sense to combine all the available tools so the Arch Mede version incorporates a faces pain scale with pain descriptors, numerical scale (0–4) and colour analogue scale (green–red: see the ONE resource) as well as the facility to individualise a tool to a child's needs.

Will Una be able to understand how to use the tool? It is really important that there is a qualitative element as well as a quantitative element thus combining literacy and numeracy aspects of this pain assessment.

There is a large body of research and knowledge with regard to validity and reliability of these tools. Stanford et al. (2006) study looked at 3–6 year olds and their abilities in using self-report scales using 112 children in equal proportion of male and female, placed in 3, 4, 5, 6 year age groups using vignettes (i.e. pain pictures of cartoons depicting various scenarios, i.e. reading a book, to scraping knee, etc.) to assess varying levels of pain. They used the Faces Pain Scales Revised (FPS-R) (Bieri et al., 1990) in order to make it possible to score on a 0–10 metric. The absence of smiles and tears (as used in the Baker and Wong (1983) scale) was seen as being advantageous in that it assessed how children feel inside, not just how the face looks. They recommend that you avoid using words ' happy' and 'sad' (which have an affective element as opposed to a sensory element of the pain experience). They found that older children were able to use FPS-R better than younger children, where 40% of 5–6 year olds really struggled to understand and use it. Whilst this study is not without its criticisms in terms of validity and reliability it offers a useful guide in terms of how children of different ages understand scales and how to explain them to children thus attending to quantitative and qualitative aspects of pain assessment and the pain experience in general. Use of number in research will be discussed in Chapter 8 in greater depth and detail.

Una appeared to understand and managed to use Arch Mede pain scale well and both she and mum were well prepared for surgery the following week, which led to an uneventful admission and postoperative recovery following surgery. Una's discharge prescription of analgesics will be discussed in other chapters.

CONCLUSION

This chapter has offered a rationale with regard to why we, as nurses, might have anxieties about our numeracy skills and has also identified where we are likely to make errors when working with number. Having defined these potential misconceptions and by developing our knowledge of number by starting from the basics, we can now start improving our skill in application of numbers as part of nursing activity. This will also help us work with children, young people and parents/carers who may have problems with numeracy skills themselves.

It is now time to reflect on your action plan before proceeding to the next chapter, which focuses on the use of numbers in counting and measuring in children and young people's nursing practice.

Chapter 2

COUNTING AND MEASURING

Numeracy in Children's Nursing, First Edition. Arija Parker
© 2015 John Wiley & Sons, Ltd. Published 2015 by John Wiley & Sons Ltd.

LEARNING FOCUS

Counting and measuring in children and young people's nursing practice

The broad focus of this chapter is on starting to define the meaning of numbers as symbols and to acquaint you with the language of numbers so that you can create your own meanings and understandings of this numeracy language. This is all set within the context of how we use numbers and symbols in nursing and healthcare settings to count and measure.

LEARNING OUTCOMES

By the end of this chapter you should be able to:

- Comprehend and utilise the numeracy language and symbols that apply to the world of child healthcare practice
- Focus in on the practical aspects of measurement and counting in nursing practice by outlining how to monitor vital signs and other measures related to child healthcare accurately
- Explore the world of imperial and SI units and know how to convert from unit to unit
- Review and revise your knowledge of children's asthma management

CASE SCENARIO 2

The case scenario is based around Banita Bhaskara (age 5) who has been admitted, with an acute exacerbation of asthma, into the Accident and Emergency Unit (A&E) at Arch Mede Hospital. She is accompanied by her reception teacher. Her parents have been informed of the transfer to hospital. She did not have her inhaler and spacer at school. Her asthma, to date, has been managed by her GP and practice nurse at her local surgery with reliever (bronchodilator) inhaler via spacer, so being treated as per Step 1 of the BTS guideline on the Management of Asthma (2014) with inhaled short-acting beta agonists when needed. She has never been in hospital before and is very anxious and frightened on admission to A&E. She was very reluctant to talk to nursing staff though was able to talk in short sentences to her teacher.

She was given a nebulised bronchodilator in A&E and oxygen was continued on from paramedic interventions during the transfer in ambulance from school.

Hospital number	AMH2014-02
Ward number	A&E + transfer to Beta Ward 2

Temperature	Pulse	Blood pressure	Respirations	CRT	Oxygen saturations	PEWS
37.4°C	130 bpm	$\frac{110}{50}$	32 per minute	1–2 seconds	92% in air	1

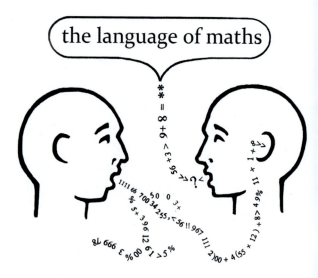

INTRODUCTION

This chapter will take a tour of the world of numbers as used in day–to-day practical nursing activities, focusing in on the numbers used when caring for Banita in the initial assessment and triage phase in the form of counting and measurement of vital signs, which are then taken a step further when she is admitted to the ward for a further 24 hours. The core discussion areas around numeracy in general will be:

- What are numbers?
- What is the metric system (including SI units and conversions)?
- What (and why) do we count and measure in children's nursing practice?

All the measures will be put into the context of counting and measuring in nursing practice using many examples that are not exclusively relevant to Banita's experiences.

SETTING THE CONTEXT

The NMC (2010) in their standards for Pre-registration Nursing Education (Essential Skills Clusters (ESC) 9 – Organisational aspects of care) require that a nurse in training:

'Accurately undertakes and records a baseline assessment of weight, height, temperature, pulse, respiration and blood pressure using manual and electronic devices' (NMC, 2010, p. 113) and also 'Measures and documents vital signs under supervision and responds appropriately to findings outside the normal range' (NMC, 2010, p. 114).

This chapter will explore all aspects of these competency requirements for student nurses and for registered nurses, who are mentoring students and also teaching these measurement skills to students, children and parents/carers also.

With regard to accurate documentation, all children at Arch Mede Hospital have patient identification bands applied not just when admitted as an inpatient. Banita had temporary name bands applied (no NHS/hospital number available initially) in A&E. The NPSA (2005) produced guidance to reduce the errors made with patient identification which was followed up in 2007 with further advice, including the following:

1. To only include the following core patient identifiers on wristbands:
   - last name
   - first name
   - date of birth
   - NHS Number (if the NHS Number is not immediately available, a temporary number should be used until it is)
2. To develop clear and consistent processes identifying which staff can produce, apply and check patient wristbands.
3. To only use a white wristband with black text, though there should be the option to have patient identifiers where there are cases of allergies using red wristbands with black text.
4. Ideally all wristbands should be generated by a centralised patient administration IT system.

This is all designed to reduce errors with patient identification where the role of numbers is key to produce unique information, that is, dates of birth and hospital numbers linked to name. Banita has both white and red patient identification bracelets applied because the teacher informed nursing staff that she is allergic to penicillin (identified from school health records).

'To use' or 'not to use' a calculator

As already stated in the preface it is worth reiterating that, whilst many nurses are totally dependent on using calculators and assessment of numeracy either at pre-registration or post-registration level **does allow** for the use of calculators, the NMC line is as follows:

The use of calculators to determine the volume or quantity of medication should not act as a substitute for arithmetical knowledge and skill. (NMC, 2007, updated 2012).

From the language used it is clear that all nurses should be able to do numeracy-related activity in relation to administration of drugs without the use of a calculator. At this stage of this chapter have a think about whether you are going to use one as your first line of calculation or whether you are going to use it just as a backup to check answers. We cannot have our numerical competence determined by whether or not we are in the possession of a calculator!

COUNTING AND USE OF WHOLE NUMBERS

It is worth starting this discussion by considering that children develop an intuitive understanding of whole numbers in relation to counting objects (see Chapter 7). So we have this innate skill from an early age where, from there, we can then develop an appreciation of how whole numbers behave, develop an understanding of place value and the patterns that are created as a result. Whilst the discussion here is not around what children are able to do in relation to number, this sets the scene well, because all our numeracy learning starts in childhood. This then allows us to really reflect on and think about how numbers guide our practise and the place of counting skills within this practice context. Clearly we can all count but how accurately do we need to be able to do this and when should we be doing it?

It is also worth remembering that not all children learn to count in the same way using numbers and language descriptions. For example, Korean children will learn using the Chisenbop finger counting method to count from 0 to 99. This is based on an abacus method.

You may also be aware of ways of learning times tables (6–10 times tables) using your fingers.

Examples and further information can be found on the website (ONE) in Section 4.

Counting on play

Counting is a really important skill that we can use to distract and play with children.

1. Young children love nursery rhymes and counting games so a repertoire of these should be part of our children's nursing toolkit that is,

   One, two, three, four, five,

   Once I caught a fish alive,

   Six, seven, eight, nine ten

   Then I let it go again

   Why did I let it go?

   Because it bit my finger so

   Which finger did it bite?

   This little finger on my right

   A favourite with many parents and children and a simple and easy way for all those who work with children to distract, amuse and build relationships with young children especially.

2. With respect to Banita, prior to discharge we will need to teach her and her mum how to use her inhaler effectively. Part of this process involves

counting and it is not easy to explain how to assemble pressurised metered-dose inhaler (PMDI) and spacer, breathe out, place mouthpiece of spacer in mouth, press inhaler once, take a slow breath in and then hold breath for 10 seconds. It is a complex technique which needs explaining at Banita's 5-year-old level of understanding, whilst also using play, trying to make it a fun thing to do! This is made more complex because of the language barriers that exist when communicating with her mother who speaks very little English, so actions and demonstration are essential, with both Banita and Mrs Bhaskara in the teaching session together.

Have a look in Section 4 for some links to nursery song and number play activity websites.
Asthma UK is a good link to 'how to use your inhaler' http://www.asthma.org.uk/how-we-help/teachers-and-healthcare-professionals/health-professionals/interactive-inhaler-demo/

The heart of nursing activity – monitoring vital signs

Accurate counting is an integral part of monitoring both respirations and pulse (heart) rate so the discussion will start with these skills.

Counting respirations

- **How to count a respiratory rate and why we do this?**

A respiratory problem is the most common reason for illness in children, particularly in the under 5 age group, as reflected by the case scenarios utilised in this book. In addition to a detailed assessment of appearance and position of the child, we need to be able to assess and count the respiratory rate of a child as accurately as possible, taking into account the external variables that will have an impact on this measure, that is, raised temperature, pain, fear and anxiety amongst others.

- **How to do it?**

Whilst it may be obvious to say it, you need to have access to a watch or clock with a second hand to be able to record a respiratory rate.

The child needs to be at rest and unaware of the fact that you are counting his or her respiratory rate, so either use some distraction, or appear to be monitoring pulse rate whilst counting respiratory rate (Kelsey and McEwing, 2008).

You need to observe the rise and fall of the child's chest, where for an infant it is easier to see this by removing clothing, though do remember not to expose the infant for any longer than you need to. Older children may not be happy to remove clothes. It is also useful to put your hand on the chest or abdomen to make it easier to count. Also, because young children are abdominal breathers it is often easier to observe the abdomen rather than chest movements (RCN, 2007).

Count the number of rise and falls (one cycle) over 60 seconds (1 minute). The commonly performed time-saving approach of counting over 15 seconds and multiplying by 4 is not an acceptable shortcut to this task, because you will not record an accurate breath per minute recording (so increasing the probability of error). Whilst you are counting you will also be observing colour, respiratory effort and rhythm, thus outlining what a complex skill this seemingly simple counting activity is when we first learn it as student nurses and when we are teaching these skills to parents or young people themselves.

Normal ranges.

Age (in years)	Respiration rate (breaths per minute)
<1	30–40
1–2	25–35
2–5	25–30
5–12	20–25
>12	15–20

Source: Mackway-Jones et al. (2005)

Auscultation, which involves listening in with a stethoscope, will increase the accuracy of the count as well as allow for more detailed assessment of the quality of breathing. This certainly helps to count respiratory rate with younger children and in Banita's case will allow you to listen for the sounds of breathing and evidence of an expiratory wheeze, if not already audible.

Counting a pulse or heart rate

- **How to count pulse and heart rates and why we do this?**

As with respiratory rates there are many external factors that need to be taken into account when measuring a pulse or heart rate including fear and anxiety, external temperature (as well as internal temperature).

Age (in years)	Heart rate (beats per minute)
<1	110–160
1–2	110–150
2–5	95–140
5–12	80–120
>12	60–100

Source: Mackway-Jones et al. (2005)

The method for doing is, most commonly, to find the radial pulse and count the rate, using a watch or clock with second hand, for a full 60 seconds (1 minute). The radial pulse can be difficult to locate in under 1's so it is easier to use the brachial artery pulse. For children under the age of 2 the RCN (2007) recommend the use of a stethoscope to count the apex beat. Please also remember that as nurses we should not rely on electronic monitoring equipment alone, that is pulse oximeters, to measure pulse rates. They should always be checked manually using palpation and/or auscultation to reduce the risk of errors.

As with respiratory rate you will also check for the quality of pulse – is it regular or irregular – is it strong or weak/thread – are there any extra beats?

Pulse force can be graded using numerical scales. (See Section 3 on ONE)

COUNTING AND MEASURING TIME

Time does not fit in with the denary (metric) system of managing numbers. This can cause all sorts of problems with calculations in nursing practice for some people so it is appropriate to deal with this issue first.

Time is based on the Babylonian system and has never been questioned or changed over time, though the French did try to decimalise it in the 1790s by having a day divided into 10 hours, each containing 100 minutes, which each had 100 seconds. Needless to say it failed dismally, because an hour with 100 minutes is not as convenient as an hour with 60 minutes, because you can divide 100 by 2, 4, 5, 10, 20, 25 and 50, but 60 can be divided by 2, 3, 4, 5, 6, 10, 12, 15, 20 and 30. This makes the units of time much easier to work with (Bellos, 2010), though can confuse us when calculating with time and other units that are measured using the metric system, that is, particularly when calculating drip rates. In children's nursing calculating drip and drop rates is not something we have to do very often though we should know how to do it.

Time is very important in how we manage our nursing routines and the routines of children we are caring for. You may have noticed that most children and young people no longer wear watches, because time is so easily accessible in digital formats such as mobile phones, though we, as nurses, do still wear a fob watch to ensure we can count pulse rates and respiratory rates.

So what units are we working with in time scales?

- 60 seconds = 1 minute
- 60 minutes = 1 hour (hr, h)
- 24 hours = 1 day (d)
- 7 days = 1 week (wk)
- 52 weeks = 1 year (yr)

And to define time-related terminology further:

- AM = ante meridiem = before midday
- PM = post meridiem = after midday

Using AM and PM or the 24-hour clock?

Use of 24-hour clock is usually used in healthcare environments so rather than writing 2 PM on a prescription chart we would usually write 14.00 hours. Have a look at the examples below and have a go at the practice questions.

AM/PM	24-hour clock
2 AM	02.00 hrs
12 midday	12.00 hrs
2 PM	14.00 hrs
8 PM	20.00 hrs
12 midnight	24.00 hrs

We also refer to parts of minutes, hours and days, that is, ½ hour = 30 minutes (go to Chapter 4 to find out more about fractions).

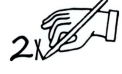

- How many seconds are there in 7 minutes?
- How many minutes are equal to 1¼ hours?
- You leave the ward to go down to pharmacy to collect Banita's take-home medications at 13.25 hours and return at 14.02. How long were you away from the ward?
- Banita is due in X-ray at 14.15 hours. It is now 13.25 and it takes 12 minutes to get to X-ray in a timely manner. At what time do you need to set off with Banita?

From the focus on counting skills in relation to pulse and respiratory rate and the discussion of how time fits into this process we now need to proceed to explore the denary/decimal/metric system which has already been discussed in Chapter 1, though now can be placed with the context of system of SI units we routinely use in our daily lives and in nursing practice.

SI UNITS – WEIGHTS AND MEASURES

SI is the abbreviation of the French 'le Système Intenational d'Unités' which was adopted worldwide in the 1960s, though whose history goes back to the 1700s in France. In the Online Dictionary it is defined as 'a complete metric system of units of measurement for scientists; fundamental quantities are length (metre) and mass (kilogram) and time (second) and electric current (ampere) and temperature (kelvin) and amount of matter (mole) and luminous intensity (candela)'.

The only country not to subscribe to this international system is the United States of America, which is of significance for European nurses who may wish to work in the United States of America and so need a knowledge of the imperial system.

To expand on the numeracy language used in the earlier chapter here are some of the prefixes we use to indicate the value of numbers.

Prefix	Meaning
Mega	Millions – some drugs are supplied in mega units – give examples
Milli	Thousandth of a unit
Micro	Millionth of a unit
Nano	Thousand-millionth of a unit

Clearly the range is from large units to very small units and some that are rarely used in practice. In children's nursing practice we use grams, milligrams and micrograms and litres and millilitres routinely so we need to be able to convert between these units with comfort.

Many nurses struggle to remember how to convert between units. What follows is advice and practice examples, which are supplemented by more worksheets and presentations on the website (ONE) Section 2.

One way to remember how to convert units is to think of size!

Small unit to **large** unit = divide (÷) i.e. 1000 mg to kg
= divide by 1000 = 1 kg (÷)

Large unit to **small** unit = multiply (×) i.e. kg to mg
= multiply by 1000 = 1000 mg (×)

Remember that if you are converting from micrograms to grams you will have to divide by 1000 twice – micrograms to milligrams (divide by 1000) and then milligrams to grams (divide by 1000) to get a final answer though this type of conversion is usually only used in tests and for practice – this activity would not be used in practice when calculating medication.

The other way of thinking about it is around the use of the decimal point and the direction you need to move it to either divide or multiply – left or right? So think – which direction?

To convert 1500 mg to grams you need to divide by 1000 and move the decimal point three places to the **LEFT** ←

1500 mg; <u>one</u> decimal place to the left ←150 (divide by 10); <u>two</u> decimal place to left ← 15 (divide by 100); <u>three</u> decimal places to the left ← 1.5 (divide by 1000) = 1.5 g

To convert 3.5 milligrams to micrograms you need to multiply by 1000 and move the decimal point three places to the **RIGHT** →

3.5 mg; <u>one</u> decimal place to the right → 35 (multiply by 10); <u>two</u> decimal places to the right → 350 (multiply by 100); <u>three</u> decimal places to the right → 3500 (multiply by 1000) = 3500 micrograms.

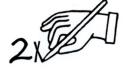

Convert the following:

675 milligrams to kilograms

1.01 kilograms to milligrams

75 milligrams to micrograms

15 micrograms to milligrams

When working with abbreviations in relation to units we do not add the 's' to the end, that is, 100 milligrams should be written as a 100 mg **not** 100 mgs.

Measuring length, height and head circumference

This is a very important measure in children's nursing practice when monitoring growth and development, which is particularly important in the early years. It is measured in metres, centimetres and millimetres. Please note that there are 10 mm in 1 cm and 100 cm in 1 metre and 1000 metres in a kilometre.

Have a go at the length conversion worksheet (Activity 2 C) on the website.

- **How to measure infants, children and young people?**

Infants are usually measured using a measuring mat so it is important that it is laid out on a solid, flat and even surface. You will need two nurses or nurse and parent to measure accurately. The infant should be lying flat with head facing up to ceiling (be careful not to hyper extend head and neck). The infant's head should touch the top of the mat and feet should be flat against the bottom with the body in a straight alignment. Visually record and then document the length on the correct centile chart. The same principles apply to an older child though clearly they will have their height measured vertically not horizontally.

The best way to learn how to perform these skills accurately is to watch the demonstration videos produced by the RCPCH: http://www.rcpch.ac.uk/child-health/research-projects/uk-who-growth-charts/uk-who-growth-chart-resources/uk-who-growth-char

The Broselow tape uses the height or length of a child to estimate weight and is a really clever, colour-coded method to get the information required particularly in a resuscitation situation.

Measuring head circumference

Head circumference is an indicator of brain growth and is a routine part of screening process up to the age of 2 years as one of the three measures recorded on a centile chart. The infant should be lying supine and then a tape measure, which is designed for the job is stretched over the occipital, parietal and frontal prominences. The average head circumference is 35 cm at birth and rapidly increases to 47 cm by the age of 1. The rate of growth then slows, reaching an average of 55 cm by the age of 6.

Interesting facts about height:

- In the first year of life children grow approximately 25 cm if born at full term
- From the age of 1–2 they grow approximately 13 cm
- From the age of 2–3 they grow approximately 9 cm per year – children typically double their birth height by the time they are 4 years old
- From the age of 3 to puberty children grow about 5 cm per year though clearly during the pubertal phase growth is erratic and is dependent on when growth spurts happen, when they can grow up to 12 cm in a year

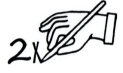

Predict Banita's height at the age of 9 by using the information above starting with a birth length of 49 cm.

VOLUME

Volume is measured in litres and millilitres though can also be measured in cubic metres. Gases like oxygen and liquids are generally measured in litres and millilitres.

1 litre = 1000 millilitres;
1 L = 1000 mL (in abbreviated form)

In children's nursing practice we use volume as a measure in many instances including measuring fluid input and output and measuring much smaller volumes when administering medications in liquid/solution form. In relation to respiratory care Banita's spacer, which is used with her PMDI to help her develop and maintain an effective technique (NICE, 2002), has a volume of 750 mL. We use them because it is really difficult for adults, never mind children, to use a PMDI alone. The skill of coordinating the pressing of the PMDI and inspiration is a complex skill. The use of a spacer allows for more time for Banita to breathe in the total amount of the metered dose of medication. The volume of the spacer is important and is dependent on the size of child and child's respiratory flow, which will also determine whether face mask or mouthpiece should be used. Spacers come in various sizes from small- to large-volume devices.

The abbreviated form of litre, which should be used, though is not always used, is a capital 'L' not lower case 'l' – why do you think this is?

When measuring out a liquid or measuring fluid amounts a meniscus will form – remember to take the reading from the bottom of the curve not the top.

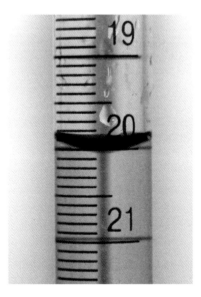

WEIGHT

The SI unit of weight is the kilogram, of which the smaller units are grams, milligrams, micrograms and nanograms.

Converting between units.

Kilogram	Gram	Milligram
1 kg	1000 g	1000000 mg
0.5 kg	500 g	500000 mg
0.1 kg	100 g	100000 mg

As already mentioned earlier on to convert from a large unit such as 1 kg to smaller units like grams you need to multiply by 1000 and to move the other way from smaller units like milligrams to large units like grams you divide by 1000.

- **How to weigh a child/young person?**

You need to ensure that you use scales suitable for the age of the child, that is, dependent on developmental age and whether they are able to sit unsupported. It is vitally important to ensure that scales calibrated correctly and that you know how to use them. Errors have been well reported via the NPSA (2007) which can lead to major medication errors. It is good practice to also double check by estimating a child's weight by using a formula (see below). Child under the age of 3 should be weighed with no clothing on (RCN, 2006) whilst, trying to persuade the child to be as still as possible which is not always easy.

It could be argued that there should not be a place for estimation in nursing practice though the opposite is true. Before you start calculating a weight or any calculation at all, it is always useful to observe the child and use a common sense approach so you have some idea of what a sensible answer should be (Hutton and Gardner, 2005).

Weight is such an important measure in children's nursing practice because most dosages are calculated on the basis of a child's weight.

When calculating weight there are two formulae commonly discussed in texts relating to the emergency care of children and young people.

1. The Resuscitation Council (UK) formula is
   (Age + 4) × 2

This is used because it is quick and easy to use in an emergency setting.

The Resuscitation Council uses this simple formula stating that complex calculations may provide greater absolute accuracy but they increase the risks for error. Drug calculations can be altered subsequently depending on further information such as actual weight or length and the response to initial treatment.

They also argue that 'pinpoint' accuracy is not essential because there are many other factors that impact the plasma levels of drugs such as body mass, method of drug administration as well as others.

2. The ILCOR/ALSG weight calculations are as follows:

Age	Formula
1–12 months	(0.5 × age months) + 4
1–5 years	(2 × age years) + 8
6–12 years	(3 × age years) + 7

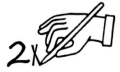

Calculate Banita's weight based on both versions of the formula.

Weight in imperial units

If for any reason you need to convert from metric to imperial units the following information is useful. We still utilise stones and pounds in day–to-day conversations about weight and most parents will know and have a better understanding of their child's weight in pounds and ounces.

Measure of weight	Equivalent weight
1 stone	14 pounds
1 pound	16 ounces
1 kg	2.2 pounds

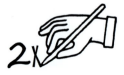

Have a go at the following conversion:

When asked about Banita's birth weight, her mum tells you that she weighed 6 pounds and 6 ounces at birth. What is her weight in kilograms?

Interesting facts about weight:

- At 2 weeks an infant regains her birth weight and then gains 0.7–0.9 kg per month
- At 3 months they gain about 500 g per month
- At 5 months they have doubled their birth weight
- At 1 year they have tripled their birth weight and gained about 200 g per month
- At 2 years they have quadrupled their birth weight and gained between 1.8–2.3 kg per year
- At the age of 9–10 they begin to gain weight faster due to onset of puberty at approximately 4.5 kg per year

Note: Please note the use of the language of maths in the use of terms like doubled, tripled, quadrupled – are these cardinal or ordinal numbers?

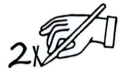

Using Banita's weight, as calculated from the conversion from pounds to kilograms, calculate her weight at the age of 5 using the lower end of the approximations.

Literacy advice in relation to prescriptions – relative errors when using weight: Which units to work in? That is, Digoxin should be prescribed in micrograms, that is, 125 micrograms not milligrams, where if it is written as 0.125 mg you can see where errors might occur due to the introduction of zero and a decimal point. Also remember that the word 'microgram' should be written in full and not be shortened to 'mcg' on a prescription chart.

SURFACE AREA

Surface area is quite a common measurement in relation to children, where some medicines may need to be calculated on the basis of body surface area (BSA). We usually use formulas or nomograms to calculate the BSA of a child or adult. It will be measured in metres squared (m^2) because you are measuring area. Advice on how to calculate square root is offered in Chapter 4.

$$\text{BSA} = \sqrt{\frac{\text{Weight (in kg)} \times \text{Height (in cm)}}{3600}}$$

This is called the Mosteller method.

Average measures of BSA for different ages.

Age of child	BSA (m^2)
Neonate	0.25
Child (age 2)	0.5
Child (age 9)	1.07
Child (age 10)	1.14
Young person/adolescent	1.33

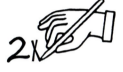

This is an extension activity which you may want to return to after reading Chapters 3 and 4. Go to a BNF for children to look at the tables at the back of the formulary that allow you to calculate BSA without needing a height measurement using the Boyd equation (BNFC, 2013).

Work out Banita's surface area using the various methods outlined to calculate it – did you get some concordance? Use her height as 106 cm and weight as 17.5 kg. You can then see whether this information fits neatly in the average BSA values cited above.

Note: You will need to use a calculator to calculate the square root of these complex numbers.

USE OF SYMBOLS – PI, ANGLES, TIME

There are many other symbols that are you are probably aware of though in the context of nursing numeracy skills do not justify particular attention in this chapter. Some of these are Pi (relating to circles), which we do not need to use in nursing practice, and angles (relating to triangles primarily), which have some relevance when needing to look at degrees of angulations (when caring for children with fractures or who may be on traction) though this is only raised as a point of interest in this book. For those of you who are interested in finding out more have a read of Enzensberger's (2000) book 'The Number Devil', which explores the importance of numbers and their relationship to triangles in a very readable and fascinating way. It is a children's book so it is visually entertaining and funny.

TEMPERATURE

This used to be measured in degree Fahrenheit and now is measured in degree Centigrade using a variety of measurement devices including mercury thermometers (no longer used in nursing practice in the UK due to the hazards of mercury and glass), tympanic thermometer, digital thermometers, using a variety of routes, though the oral and rectal route should not be used routinely for children from 0 to 5 years of age (NICE, 2007). As already discussed it is vitally important to be able to use the equipment, that is, thermometers in this case, accurately and correctly. The advantages of using a tympanic thermometer with children is the speed of recording though inaccuracies can arise due to poor technique. At Arch Mede Hospital they use tympanic thermometers as guided by evidence from the RCN (2007) which recommends that infants under the age of 4 weeks to 5 years have an electronic/chemical dot thermometer or an infrared tympanic thermometer used. Whatever the method of measurement it is vitally important that temperature is measured for the correct length of time to gain an accurate reading.

As with pulse and respiratory rate measurement there will be variations due to factors such as time of day, exercise, age and environmental factors that may need to be taken into account. Where nurses are caring for the very young they will need to manage environmental temperatures to maintain the comfort of their patients in relation to the activities of living and especially when bathing and washing as one example of many.

Temperature measurement – Fahrenheit or Celsius?

The Fahrenheit temperature scale was proposed by physicist Daniel Gabriel Fahrenheit in 1724. The scale was based on three reference points which are the freezing point of water, the temperature of the human body and the boiling point of water. It is still used in the United States of America though most countries now use degree Centigrade. The Celsius scale was developed by Anders Celsius in 1742 and is a scale of temperature in which 0° represents the melting point of ice and 100° represents the boiling point of water. Measurement in the Kelvin system is used mainly in science.

If interested in using formulae have a go at converting between Fahrenheit and Celsius!

$$^{\circ}C \times 9/5 + 32 = {^{\circ}F}$$

$$(^{\circ}F - 32) \times 5/9 = {^{\circ}C}$$

Normal ranges of temperature for different thermometers

Site of measurement	Range in °C
Tympanic	36.9–37.5
Axilla	35.8–36.6
Oral	36.4–37.4
Rectal	37–37.8

PRESSURE

The SI unit for pressure is Pascal (Pa) which is named after a French physicist and mathematician Blaise Pascal. This is the unit used to measure blood gases though it is expressed usually in kilopascals (KPa), it is also measured in millimetres of mercury (mmHg) which we most ordinarily understand in nursing practice as a measure of blood pressure.

What is Blood Pressure?

Blood pressure is the force per unit area exerted on the wall of a blood vessel by the blood it contains (Marieb, 1999). It is measured in millimetres of mercury – mmHg, because the measuring devices used are manometers (which are instruments that measure pressure with the height of a column of liquid), that is, sphygmomanometers. Mercury is used because it means that the instruments used can be smaller. If water was used the manometer would be over 3 metres tall.

When the heart contracts, blood is ejected from the ventricles into the aorta and the pulmonary arteries under very high pressure. This pressure averages 120 mmHg in adults who are healthy, though this obviously varies and is dependent on age in our younger patients (see normal ranges below). This pressure gradually declines throughout the rest of the circulatory system until the blood returns to the heart in the right atrium where the pressure has dropped to 0 mmHg.

After contraction or systole, the heart enters its relaxation phase or diastole. At this point the pressure in the aorta drops to its lowest level, approximately 70–80 mmHg in adults. This is the diastolic pressure.

This is why you see the blood pressure written down as two figures as follows:

100 Systolic

60 Diastolic

So to summarise, the systolic blood pressure reflects the pressure in the arteries when the heart is contracting and the diastolic pressure is the pressure in the arteries when the heart is at rest.

When measuring any vital signs it is important to be aware of the range of normal values. From experience there is no such thing as normal blood pressure as it can vary greatly between one person and another. However a normal range for an adult may be from 100/60 to 150/90. The term for high blood pressure is hypertension, and for low blood pressure hypotension.

Normal ranges of blood pressure for different age groups.

Age (in years)	Systolic BP in mmHg
<1	70–90
1–2	75–95
2–5	85–100
5–12	90–110
>12	100–120

It is important to note that performing blood pressures on very young children can be difficult to do and we do not always monitor blood pressure routinely in all children for this reason, though clearly in an emergency situation, where a child is acutely unwell, we do monitor BP.

Before we consider how to actually take a blood pressure there is an important concept to consider when performing a manual BP. What are we actually listening to and measuring?

The Korotkoff sounds are described in five phases:

Phase 1: Level at which the first clear tapping sounds are heard. This represents the systolic blood pressure

Phase 2: Blowing or swishing sounds

Phase 3: Sharp, but softer sounds than in 1

Phase 4: Sound becomes muffled

Phase 5: Sound disappears – this is the diastolic blood pressure

There is debate on whether diastolic should be measured at phase 4 or 5, however the recommendations of the British Hypertension Society is to measure it at stage 5.

The two main ways of measuring blood pressure are:

- Indirectly by the use of electronic monitoring systems. A cuff is attached to the child's arm, which is inflated automatically by the machine. It is then displayed on the machine as two readings, the systolic and the diastolic.
- Manually, using a stethoscope and mercury sphygmomanometer. Although most hospitals rely on electronic readings of blood pressure it is important that as a nurse you are able to measure the blood pressure manually. In low reading hypotension, less than 70 mmHg it can be almost impossible to get a reading from an electronic machine, and you may have to resort to a manual reading, where you can only get a systolic reading. As a general rule of thumb if you can feel a radial pulse then the systolic blood pressure is 80 mmHg or above. If there is no radial pulse the systolic is less than 70 mmHg (taking account that this is very approximate rule of thumb).

As reflected in NMC (2010) standards, there is a requirement that children's nurses are able to perform both manual and electronic blood pressure on various ages of children.

Whether using electronic measuring devices or manual it is very important to get the correct cuff size. The cuff consists of an inflatable bladder within a restrictive cloth sheath. It is the dimensions of the bladder within the sheath that affect the accuracy of blood pressure measurement. The bladder length should be at least 80% of the circumference of the limb to which it is to be applied. If the bladder is too small overestimation of blood pressure will occur and conversely if it is too large underestimation of blood pressure. There are usually some reference marks on the cuff to avoid making mistakes with cuff size. The cuff should also not be too narrow.

Cuff sizes in relation to size (infant to adult).

Size	Measurement in cm
Small infant	7–10
Infant	9–13
Small child	12–16
Child	15–21
Small adult	20–26
Adult	25–34

Please note that the sizes vary dependent on the manufacturer of the cuff, so it is vitally important to ensure that you are clear about which cuff you should use, which will involve measuring a child's arm to get the correct cuff size or visually checking that the bladder encircles at least 80% of the arm. It should also be applied with the centre of the bladder over the brachial artery. The child should be seated, the arm supported at the level of the heart with no tight clothes restricting the arm whether using an electronic monitoring device or a sphygmomanometer.

The fifth vital sign – pain assessment

This has been discussed in Chapter 1 and is an integral part of monitoring vital signs and is viewed as the fifth vital sign (RCN, 2009). Banita did have a pain assessment recorded as part of her triage and scored '0' – no pain at all. Numerical pain scales vary from 0–4, 0–5, 0–10.

Part of your PDP plan could be to consider why the numbers and scale is important.

CHARTING COUNTING AND MEASUREMENT

This final section of Chapter 2 will outline some of the documentation used to record our findings, Paediatric Early Warning Scores (PEWS), some further skills used to assess our patients as well as the numbers that relate to the care of Banita and her family.

The move beyond TPR/BP alone on a chart to integrate other observations into a system of PEWS

Defining paediatric early warning scores

Adult-orientated early warning scores (which are called by various names) have been in place since the late 1990s motivated by the need to detect deterioration in the condition of patients earlier rather than later, through the concept of 'critical care without walls' (DOH, 2000). This has also been taken on-board in children's care settings in the form of PEWS (also called by various names).

NICE (2007a) produced guidelines aimed at reducing the risk for acutely ill patients using a 'track and trigger' system to measure, record and act on patients' physiological status measured via vital sign measurement. The aim is to track the progress of all patients and trigger an immediate response should the warning score indicate the need.

The reason we have a paediatric version of these charts is that physiologically changes happen in a different way dependent on age, within a different range of parameters where children tend to deteriorate more rapidly in an acute situation. Often PEWS charts will cover different age ranges on different charts rather than using a single chart alone. In general, all patients have their vital signs measured and, depending on the shaded areas identified on these charts, these are converted into a colour-coded risk band, which is documented on the front of the observation chart. The nearer to the red risk band the more abnormal the vital signs are. If the measurements reach above a certain threshold a doctor must be called to assess the patient. The system allows for the regular monitoring and recording of blood pressure, pulse, temperature, Glasgow Coma Score (GCS), Alert, Voice, Pain, Unresponsive (AVPU), urine output and respiratory rate on adult charts.

On children's PEWS charts the usual observations of TPR/BP as well as respiratory distress, oxygen saturation and conscious level are recorded. These do vary from hospital to hospital, though the principles are the same. No consensus exists with how the charts should look or be used and a simplified form is illustrated below. Other areas will use shading in observation charts rather than a table as in this Arch Mede Hospital format (which accompanies the observation chart). The charts on ONE have shading identifying normal ranges of the vital signs making them easier to interpret. The charts offer a detailed way of recording a lot of numerical information.

Arch Mede PEWS chart.

	3	2	1	0	SCORE
Cardiovascular	Grey and mottled OR CRT ≥OR Tachycardia (30 above normal for age) OR bradycardia (dependent on age)	Grey OR CRT 4 seconds OR Tachycardia (20 above normal for age)	Pale OR CRT 3 seconds	Pink OR CRT 1–2 seconds	
Respiratory	5 below normal range with sternal recession, tracheal tug or grunting AND/OR 50% FiO_2 or 8 + litres/min (if high-flow face mask being used)	>20 above normal parameters Using accessory muscles, 40% FiO_2 Oxygen ≥3 Lpm	>10 above normal parameters Using accessory muscles, 30% FiO_2 Any initiation of oxygen	Normal limits for age No recession or abnormal signs SaO_2 is above 92% in air	

(continued)

	3	2	1	0	SCORE
Behaviour	Lethargic, confused OR reduced pain response	Irritable OR agitated and not consolable	Sleeping	Playing Appropriate behaviour for this child	
Please note: Score 2 extra for ½ hourly nebulisers or persistent vomiting following surgery					
				TOTAL	

Arch Mede Hospital developed their early warning score based on the one developed by the adult areas and then by sharing good practice within the paediatric network, which meets on a monthly basis. Whilst there is no standard PEWS approach in place within all hospitals which care for children, the approach used is reviewed on an annual basis to ensure that it is a tool that does what it is meant to do in terms of trigger for the correct reason, that is, early detection of deterioration of an acutely ill child.

NHS Institute innovation and improvement – to get more information about the use of PEWS and access different examples of the charts that can be used.
http://www.institute.nhs.uk/safer_care/paediatric_safer_care/pews.html

At Arch Mede Hospital the following actions are triggered by the scores as below:

1   Continue routine observations
2   Inform the senior nurse who is coordinating and leading the shift
3   On call doctor to be informed and to attend within 30 minutes
4   **or above** – Inform senior nurse, doctor on call to attend within 15 minutes, registrar (more senior doctor) to attend, inform consultant, repeat observations after 15 minutes. If score remains the

same after four sets of recordings move to high
dependency area and monitor 1:1.

**At all stages ensure that records are kept contemporaneously
to ensure accuracy.**

All bed end folders for children also include normal
observations for the different age groups as outlined earlier
in this chapter so that nurse do not need to memorise
this information (though all should know what the normal
ranges for children as an estimate).

Defining the terms used on the PEWS chart

1.   What is FiO$_2$?

Fraction of inspired oxygen (FiO$_2$) is the fraction or
percentage of oxygen in the space being measured. FiO$_2$
is used to represent the percentage of oxygen used in
gaseous exchange (see table below for the FiO$_2$ and rates of
flow in relation to oxygen administration via Venturi mask).
The FiO$_2$ of air is 21%.

2.   What is a capillary refill time (CRT)?

Measuring capillary refill is a simple and effective way to
assess circulatory status of infants and children and is
the rate at which blood returns to the capillary bed after it
has been compressed digitally (RCN, 2007) This should
not be used as a measure in isolation of other measures,
which applies to all the vital signs it could be argued.
They come as a package – as a children's assessment toolkit!

Sites used are the skin of forehead or chest (sternum),
where pressure is applied with forefinger sufficiently to
blanch the skin. This pressure is maintained for 5 seconds
and then released and what is then measured is the time it
takes (in seconds) for the skin to return to its normal colour.
The normal perfusion rate is less than 2 seconds in children
and less than 3 seconds in neonates (RCN, 2007).

3.   What is oxygen saturation?

This is a non-invasive way of monitoring the oxygen
saturation of haemoglobin in arterial blood. The

pulse oximeters work on the principle of Beer–Lambert law which states that the concentration of an unknown solute in a solvent can be determined by light absorption and measures oxygen saturation as a percentage.

That is,

$$L \text{ (out)} = L \text{ (in)} - (DCa)$$

L = intensity of light

C = concentration of solution

D = distance the height travels through the solution

a = absorption coefficient of solute.

As already discussed it is vital that the equipment is used correctly, particularly in choosing the correct probe in relation to the child's size and the site used for monitoring. There are many reasons why inaccuracies occur, which range from movement of sensor to the presence of nail varnish and dirt, lack of haemoglobin in the blood, to name but a few. The site used needs to be warm and well perfused. Just to repeat what has already been said, as with other measurements it cannot be relied on alone as a measure and needs to be viewed within the context of other vital signs measured. The normal range is usually defined as 94–100%.

4. Why record behaviour to assess level of consciousness?

Neurological observations are performed when children are admitted with head injuries, though are also utilised when we want to quickly assess a child's level of consciousness in general, whatever the underlying pathophysiology. A quick assessment tool to use is AVPU.

- **AVPU**

Letter	Descriptor	PEW score
A	Alert	0
V	Responds to voice	1
P	Responds to pain	2
U	Unresponsive	3

Banita was triaged using AVPU in A&E and was scored at zero (0).

- **Modified GCS**

The following table reflects the key components of the assessment of level of consciousness which results with a score out of 15. This is a more refined tool than AVPU though it takes more time to complete. It was originally developed by Teasdale and Jennett (1974) though it has been adapted to suit the needs of infants and children over the years since it was first developed. We usually use a modified scale that takes into account a child's developmental stage, that is, in relation to communication – there may be problems for children with responding to direction (motor response) and verbalising, which are key components of the scale as follows:

- Eye opening
- Best verbal response
- Motor response

From evaluating these you end up with a numerical score out of 15 though then need to proceed to examine pupillary activity – size, shape, equality and reaction of pupils to light, response to painful stimuli and limb movements in much greater depth to form a thorough picture of the child's neurological status. The neurological assessment also includes measurement of vital signs as already discussed above.

The scores that trigger certain responses and activity are as follows:

- A score of 15 is the maximum score – child responsive and alert
- Lowest score possible is 3 – deep coma
- Once the score falls below 12 the child needs to be closely monitored
- Once below 8 child will need mechanical support with respiration – intubation and ventilation

It is a very sensitive scale indeed (NICE, 2007b).

Pupil size chart used at Arch Mede Hospital (not drawn to scale).

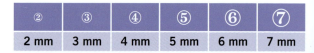

②	③	④	⑤	⑥	⑦
2 mm	3 mm	4 mm	5 mm	6 mm	7 mm

Good numeracy practice when completing charts

The links between dots on a page should be connected with straight lines not loops (or bunny hops!)

How often to monitor vital signs?

These should not be done as part of a ward routine, that is, four hourly, though should be individualised and assessed, measured and recorded as part of the initial assessment in hospital settings and then the decision made on the frequency of recording dependent on the child's status (RCN, 2007). Banita did have her respiratory rate, pulse rate, oxygen saturations, level of consciousness monitored hourly whilst in A&E and gradually, as her condition improved, they were recorded two hourly and then four hourly overnight.

Update on case scenario

Banita and family are transferred to the children's unit for further assessment and observation overnight where her condition improved following administration of oxygen for a few hours, regular nebulisers containing a bronchodilator (due to poor compliance and technique with PMDI and spacer) and oral prednisolone for 3 days.

The oxygen was administered via a Venturi mask, which is a type of disposable mask used to deliver a controlled oxygen concentration to a patient. The flow of 100% oxygen through the Venturi mask draws in a controlled amount of room air (21% oxygen). The Venturi principle works by using a tube with a decrease in the inside diameter that is used to increase the flow velocity of the fluid and thereby cause a pressure drop. With oxygen delivery systems oxygen flows through the tubing and room air is drawn in a controlled amount to regulate the amount given to the patient. The system is adaptable to different oxygen requirements as shown in the table below. Please remember that oxygen has to be prescribed.

Following discussion with parents it became clear that they did not know how to administer the preventer inhaler she had been prescribed, even though the technique had been explained by the practice nurse. There were language difficulties preventing effective communication. She was discharged home as per Step 2 of the BTS guidelines (2014) on inhaled steroids and preventer administered via spacer as required with the advice to use the preventer regularly for the next couple of days. She was also visited by the community children's nursing team to check inhaler technique and the team also talked to school about Banita's asthma management. This nurse could also talk to the mum in Gujarati as well as English, which really helped with the teaching of these skills.

Venturi mask colour coding and flow rates

Colour	Flow rate (litres/minute)	FiO$_2$
Blue	2	24
White	4	28
Orange	6	31
Yellow	8	35
Red	8	40
Green	15	60

As recommended by BTS (2014), whilst a peak expiratory flow measurement would have been useful to aid recognition of the severity of Banita's condition she has never done this before. She is only 5 and was too distressed on admission to cooperate anyway. BTS (2014) recommend that children over the age of 6 should be able to learn how to do a peak flow.

There are many types of peak flow meter, where two different types known as low and standard range are used at Arch Mede Hospital as follows:

- Standard range peak flow meters are suitable for both adults and children.
- Low range peak flow meters are designed for adults with low readings, and for children.

The better controlled the asthma the higher the peak flow score will be and these measures are used to help children and families self-manage their asthma (using diaries). They are measured in litres per minute and are relatively easy to read and record if patients are able to read and understand numbers.

A way of estimating what the peak expiratory flow rate (PEFR) should be is to use this formula (only relevant for young adults)

PEFR (L/min) = [Height (cm) − 80] × 5

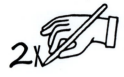

Calculate the PEFR for young people of the following heights (we cannot do it for Banita – she is not tall enough to use this calculation and too young to do it anyway):

- 110 cm
- 135 cm
- 162 cm

A much more accurate way is to use charts and nomograms. You can have a look at on these on the website where there is guidance on what peak flow meters look like and how to use one.

CONCLUDING COMMENTS

This chapter has focused in on the counting and measurement used in children's practice. It has covered most of the ways we assess and monitor children's vital signs and also looked at how important numbers are in relation to the equipment that is used in healthcare practice, in hospitals and at home. Not only do nurses need to be able to count and measure but we may also may have to teach children, young people and their families to perform these skills and monitor health-related problems at home. There are areas where more complex counting needs to be undertaken, that is, when working in intensive care environments or other specialist areas.

Your PDP activity at this stage involves reflecting on your practice context to identify how you can develop your counting skills further.

Chapter 3

. . . .

BASIC NUMERACY SKILLS UNDERPINNING CHILDREN AND YOUNG PEOPLE'S NURSING PRACTICE

Numeracy in Children's Nursing, First Edition. Arija Parker

© 2015 John Wiley & Sons, Ltd. Published 2015 by John Wiley & Sons Ltd.

LEARNING FOCUS

Basic numeracy skills
Revision (or it could be the re-learning) of how to do addition, subtraction, multiplication and division and the use of these numeracy skills in monitoring the fluid balance of children and young people.

LEARNING OUTCOMES

By the end of this chapter you should be able to:

- Evaluate your present approach to these basic numerical skills and consider alternatives that may make these skills easier to do – addition, subtraction, multiplication and division
- Review your knowledge of the care and management of a child with gastroenteritis
- Recognise the importance of accurate monitoring of fluid balance and calculate the fluid requirements for children and young people and have the numeracy know-how to be able to do this with confidence

CASE SCENARIO 3

Tommy Turing (2) has been admitted to Beta Ward 2 at Arch Mede Hospital, with gastroenteritis. He lives with mum and dad and has two older siblings – Tim (6) and Tanya (9). He has been vomiting for the past 2 days. This started whilst he was at nursery and he is now experiencing profuse diarrhoea. He is admitted to a cubicle on the ward with what appears to be mild-to-moderate dehydration. This is Tommy's first period of hospitalisation. He is fully immunised and is usually a lively and active little boy who is meeting all his developmental milestones. He was born at full term with no complications. He is now fretful, curled up on his mum's lap, with a mouth that looks very dry, having last vomited half an hour ago.

An example of observation charts and fluid balance charts for 1 day of his 3 days of hospitalisation is included in the ONE resource. His fluid balance charts and calculations in relation to fluid requirements in general, will form the basis of activities which will assess your abilities in addition, subtraction, multiplication and division as the numeracy skill focus for this chapter.

Hospital number	AMH2012-03
Ward number	Beta Ward 2 (The children's unit)

Temperature	Pulse	Blood pressure	Respirations	CRT	Pain score	PEWS
38.7°C	132 bpm	60 systolic	26 per minute	2 seconds	4 (Mum's assessment)	1

Blood results (from Day 1)

Urea and electrolytes	Tommy's results on Day 2	Normal ranges
Sodium	124 mmol/L	136–143 mmol/L
Potassium	3.8 mmol/L	4.1–5.6 mmol/L
Chloride	96 mmol/L	98–106 mmol/L
Bicarbonate	22 mmol/L	22–26 mmol/L
Creatinine	80 µmol/L	<80 µmol/L
Urea	7.1 mmol/L	2.5–6.7 mmol/L

Birth weight	Height (on admission)	Weight (on admission)	BSA (if needed)
8 lb 7 oz = 4 kg	92 cm	11.8 kg Actual weight = 12.5 kg	0.55 cm^2

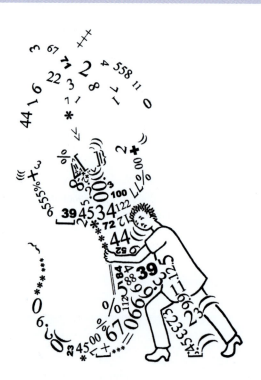

INTRODUCTION

This chapter will take us back to the basic operations we use in all numeracy activities, namely addition, subtraction, multiplication and division. Unless we achieve mastery in these skills it is difficult to progress to other areas of numeracy practice. If you are unsure about the method you presently use for these operations have a go at the different methods suggested here. It does take some time to change the habits of a lifetime, though it is worth persevering with some of these methods, particularly long multiplication if, when you first try it, this could be the method for me though it does seem more complicated than the traditional method. Many examples will be offered using whole numbers and decimals.

Please also access the ONE resource where PowerPoint presentations explain the processes.

Setting the context

The NMC (2010) in their standards for Pre-registration Nursing Education ESC 29 states that:

'People can trust a newly registered graduate nurse to assess and monitor their fluid status and in partnership with them, formulate an effective plan of care' and 'Accurately monitors and records fluid intake and output' and, at point of registration, 'Identifies signs of dehydration and acts to correct these' (NMC, 2012, p. 131).

ESC 32 states that 'People can trust the newly registered graduate nurse to safely administer fluids when fluids cannot be taken independently' and by entry to register and 'Monitors and assesses people receiving intravenous fluids' and 'Documents progress against prescription and markers of hydration' (NMC, 2010, p. 133)

This chapter will explore some of the numeracy aspects of these competency statements, thus looking at hydration status, fluid balance and the numerical aspects of parenteral therapy used when Tommy is unable to tolerate fluids orally.

The numerical operations explained

1. Addition

Addition is the mathematical process of adding and involves finding the total or sum of two or more numbers in the following fashion:

$$3 + 6 + 7 = 16$$

It follows some important patterns in that it is commutative, which means that the order of the numbers does not matter i.e. $7 + 6 + 3$ gets the same result and it is also associative in that you can group the numbers in any way also, that is, $(3 + 6) + 7 = 3 + (6 + 7) = 16$.

Just to define this new terminology a bit further. An operation is **associative** if you can group numbers in any way without changing the answer. It does not matter how you combine them, the answer will always be the same. Addition and multiplication are both associative.

An operation is **commutative** if you can change the order of the numbers involved without changing the result. Addition and multiplication are both commutative.

Addition can be done by mentally adding the numbers up as you go along or by using the following approach, especially when utilising larger numbers.

$$6786 + 5509 = ?$$

Start by lining up the numbers with due regard to place value. You will be working with the numbers from right to left starting with units and moving through tens, hundreds etc.

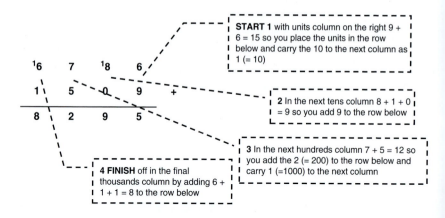

START 1 with units column on the right 9 + 6 = 15 so you place the units in the row below and carry the 10 to the next column as 1 (= 10)

2 In the next tens column 8 + 1 + 0 = 9 so you add 9 to the row below

3 In the next hundreds column 7 + 5 = 12 so you add the 2 (= 200) to the row below and carry 1 (=1000) to the next column

4 FINISH off in the final thousands column by adding 6 + 1 + 1 = 8 to the row below

When carrying the units to tens to hundreds feel free to add the numbers to top row of digits or the bottom line (as below) – it does not matter – whatever works better for you!

6	7	8	6	
^{1}1	5	^{1}0	9	+
8	2	9	5	

Now let us try numbers which include a decimal point, that is, 53·75 + 36·93. Work in the same way as above with due regard to place value and the place occupied by the decimal point.

5	3	·	7	5	
¹3	¹6	·	9	3	+
9	0	·	6	8	

Words used to define 'addition'	Symbols used to signify 'addition'
Add, Addition, Sum, Plus, Increase, Total	+

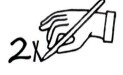

Adding numbers: Add the following numbers together

- 59 + 82 =
- 773 + 94 =
- 71189 + 3901 =
- 7.5 + 9.1 =
- 75.82 + 6.731 =
- 700.821 + 3.21 =

2. Subtraction

Subtraction is the process of taking a number away from another number resulting in a value that is the difference between two numbers and is the opposite of addition. Subtraction is not associative or commutative: 2 − 1 is not equal to 1 − 2. So the order does matter when defining the problem. If the subtraction problem is written in words, that is, take 16 away from 86, you need to read the information, guidance offered and define the subtraction problem clearly so that you get the order correct, that is, 86 − 16 = 70.

There are two methods which can be used, besides the methods you may use when maybe calculating the change you should be given when shopping where you may use a 'counting on' method for simple subtraction, that is, take 65 from 86 – count on from 65 to 70 (= 5), then from 70 to 80 (= 10) and finally from 80 to 86 (= 6), then add together $5 + 10 + 6 = 21$.

METHOD 1 – 'borrowing by adding' to bottom row of numbers – called the 'borrowing' method or 'equal addition' most commonly. You place the number that you are subtracting from on the top row and the number to be subtracted on the second row. As with addition you move from the column on the right in order to the left.

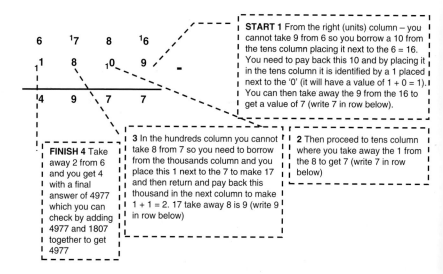

START 1 From the right (units) column – you cannot take 9 from 6 so you borrow a 10 from the tens column placing it next to the 6 = 16. You need to pay back this 10 and by placing it in the tens column it is identified by a 1 placed next to the '0' (it will have a value of 1 + 0 = 1). You can then take away the 9 from the 16 to get a value of 7 (write 7 in row below).

2 Then proceed to tens column where you take away the 1 from the 8 to get 7 (write 7 in row below)

3 In the hundreds column you cannot take 8 from 7 so you need to borrow from the thousands column and you place this 1 next to the 7 to make 17 and then return and pay back this thousand in the next column to make 1 + 1 = 2. 17 take away 8 is 9 (write 9 in row below)

FINISH 4 Take away 2 from 6 and you get 4 with a final answer of 4977 which you can check by adding 4977 and 1807 together to get 4977

METHOD 2 – 'borrowing by subtracting' from top row of numbers which is also called the 'decomposition' method

In this method you can work as in the top example but instead of borrowing from the bottom row of numbers you work in tens, hundreds and thousands and take away (subtract) from the top column.

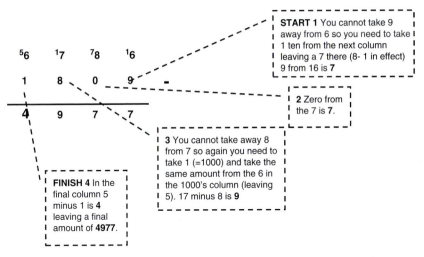

START 1 You cannot take 9 away from 6 so you need to take 1 ten from the next column leaving a 7 there (8- 1 in effect) 9 from 16 is **7**

2 Zero from the 7 is **7**.

3 You cannot take away 8 from 7 so again you need to take 1 (=1000) and take the same amount from the 6 in the 1000's column (leaving 5). 17 minus 8 is **9**

FINISH 4 In the final column 5 minus 1 is **4** leaving a final amount of **4977**.

Subtraction is all important when thinking about adding up fluid balance and identifying whether your patient is in a positive or negative balance (see below).

Subtraction with decimal point and places is exactly the same as in addition where you just maintain the place of the decimal point and work as demonstrated above.

Words used to define 'subtraction'	Symbols
Subtract, Subtraction, Minus, Less, Difference, Decrease, Take Away, Deduct	–

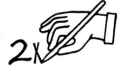

Subtracting numbers: Subtract the following numbers

- $96 - 53 =$
- $782 - 531 =$
- $632198 - 55421 =$
- $7.9 - 3.7 =$
- $77.365 - 52.92 =$
- $30621.5 - 7333.71 =$

3. Multiplication

Multiplication is the process of adding numbers many times. As with addition multiplication is both associative and commutative. Nursing students generally have major problems with what is known as 'long multiplication' so the purpose here will be to demonstrate many different methods both to illustrate how children are being taught at school, and also to give you opportunities to find a better way of performing this skill. Learning the times tables as a child appears to make it easier to do multiplications as an adult though. Sousa (2008) argues that our troubles with numbers have multifactorial problems linked with them included in associative memory, pattern recognition and language. Many of us learned times tables by rote – is this an advantage? Why do we struggle to memorise times tables when we are able to remember 10 new words every day and remember names, phone numbers, book titles, words to songs with ease in childhood? Interesting to think about.

- **Traditional method**

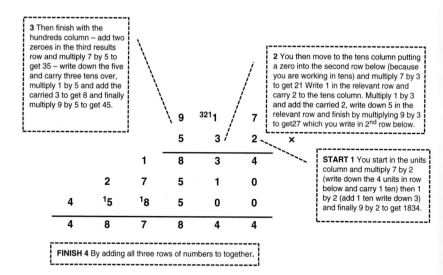

3 Then finish with the hundreds column – add two zeroes in the third results row and multiply 7 by 5 to get 35 – write down the five and carry three tens over, multiply 1 by 5 and add the carried 3 to get 8 and finally multiply 9 by 5 to get 45.

2 You then move to the tens column putting a zero into the second row below (because you are working in tens) and multiply 7 by 3 to get 21 Write 1 in the relevant row and carry 2 to the tens column. Multiply 1 by 3 and add the carried 2, write down 5 in the relevant row and finish by multiplying 9 by 3 to get27 which you write in 2nd row below.

START 1 You start in the units column and multiply 7 by 2 (write down the 4 units in row below and carry 1 ten) then 1 by 2 (add 1 ten write down 3) and finally 9 by 2 to get 1834.

FINISH 4 By adding all three rows of numbers to together.

- **Grid method**

You have been asked to multiply 917 by 530.

Step 1: Split the number into hundreds, tens and units.

i.e. 900, 10, 7 and 500, 30, 2

Step 2: Draw a grid and insert the numbers – one number horizontally and the other vertically.

Then multiply the numbers within the grid with each other.

×	900	10	7
500	450000	5000	3500
30	27000	300	210
2	1800	20	14

Step 3: Then add the numbers together either underneath the lattice or by adding a 'totals' column at the end of the grid as follows:

$$450000 + 5000 + 3500 + 27000 + 300 + 210 + 1800 + 20 + 14 = 487844$$

×	900	10	7	Totals
500	450000	5000	3500	458500
30	27000	300	210	27510
2	1800	20	14	1834
				487844

This works well with whole numbers though becomes very complex when working with numbers that need a decimal point in place though, as with other methods you can remove the decimal points and just remember to replace them when you get your final answer. As you can see with large numbers you need to have a clear understanding of place value and the use of zero as a place holder – you can see that it would be easy to make an error with the number of zeroes that are being used.

- **Lattice method**

The worked example involves multiplying 917 by 532 and you need to start by placing one number horizontally at the top of the grid and the other one vertically down the side of the grid.

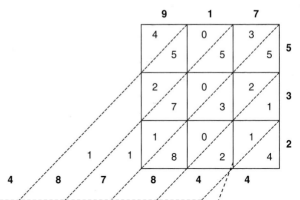

START 1 Start on the right hand side and work your way down and then across systematically. Multiply 7 by 5 = 35 and place the number in the box as shown above with the 3 in the top of the split cell and 5 in the bottom.
2 Then multiply 7 by 3 = 21 and do the same in the relevant box and carry on doing the same with the rest of the numbers. Where you have a single digit number i.e. 1 by 3 = 3 you place the number in the bottom of the split cell (which is why zero has been used as a place holder in the top of the split cell).
FINISH 3 When the grid is complete you add up along the lattice lines and where you end up with a two digit number you carry the '1' in this case) to the next lattice column to get an answer of 487844.

Have a look at ONE Section 3. There is a copy of a lattice which you could laminate and then use and reuse when practicing long multiplication using this method.

This method works well with decimal numbers where you just need to count the decimal places and place the decimal point equal to decimal places in the final answer, that is, if multiplying 9.17 by 5.32, you would have four decimal places and so the final answer would be 48.7844.

- **Vedic mathematics method**

Vedic mathematics is based on 16 sutras, presented by a Hindu mathematician Bharati Krishna Tirthaji Maharaja. The rationale for using it here is that it is a creative and exciting way of doing long multiplication and is being used to teach children long multiplication in some schools.

Using the sutra called 'vertically and horizontally' this is a different, fun and space-saving method for multiplying whole numbers.

Step 1: Write the numbers clearly lined up as in the traditional method.

$$4 \qquad 7$$

$$8 \qquad 3$$

Step 2: Multiply the digits in the right-hand column, that is, $7 \times 3 = 21$. The final digit of the answer is the last digit of the answer. Write the '1' in the right-hand column and carry the '2' as follows:

$$4 \qquad 7$$
$$\qquad \qquad 1$$
$$8 \qquad 3$$
$$\qquad \qquad {}_2 1$$

Step 3: Find the sum of the crosswise products $(4 \times 3) + (7 \times 8) = 12 + 56 = 68$. Add the 2 that is carried from the previous step to get 70. The final digit is 0, which is written in the left-hand column with 7 carried over.

$$4 \qquad 7$$

$$8 \qquad 3$$
$${}_7 0 \qquad 1$$

Step 4: Multiply the digits in the left-hand column, $4 \times 8 = 32$. Add the 7 that has been carried over to make 39 to give the final answer.

$$\qquad \qquad 4 \qquad 7$$
$$\qquad \qquad 1$$
$$\qquad \qquad 8 \qquad 3$$
$$3 \qquad 9 \qquad 0 \qquad 1$$

This method can be used with numbers of any size where with more numbers there need to be more vertically and cross-multiplied. Another example is included below, that is, 532×917 and there are many more included online as well as practice examples.

Step 1: Start with the digits in the right-hand column, that is, $2 \times 7 = 14$.

5	3	2
		|
9	1	7
		$_14$

Step 2: Sum of the cross products $(3 \times 7) + (2 \times 1) = 23$ plus the 1 that has been carried over, that is, 24. Insert the 4 in the middle column and carry the 2.

5	3	2
	×	
9	1	7
	$_24$	4

Step 3: Now we move to the cross products in the units and hundreds column and add the product of the vertical product of the tens column (centre), that is, $(5 \times 7) + (9 \times 2) + (3 \times 1) = 56$ plus the 2 that has been carried, that is, 58.

5	3	2
|		
9	1	7
$_58$	4	4

Step 4: Now we move to the cross products in the tens and hundreds column, that is, $(5 \times 1) + (3 \times 9) = 32$ to which we add the 5 that is carried over, that is, 37. We insert the 7 in the thousands column and go to the final step.

		5	3	2
		×		
		9	1	7
	₃7	8	4	4

Step 5: Finally we find the vertical product in the left hand (hundreds) column as follows, that is, $5 \times 9 = 45$ and add the 3 that has been carried over, that is, 48.

			5	3	2
			I		
			9	1	7
4	8	7	8	4	4

Multiplying with decimal point and places

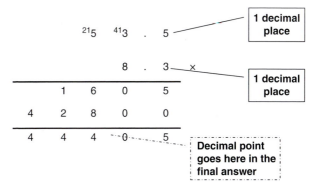

The decimal point needs to be placed in the final answer. We need to replace two decimal places so the final answer will be **444.05.**

Words used to define 'multiplication'	Symbols
Multiply, Multiplication, Product, By, Times, Lots Of	× or *

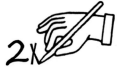

Multiplying numbers

- $55 \times 19 =$
- $621 \times 78 =$
- $8.9 \times 10 =$
- $5.5 \times 1.5 =$
- $63.3 \times 11.3 =$

Have a look at ONE Section 4 at the Chinese stick method for multiplication – good fun and a different way of multiplying especially when teaching children how to do long division. The YouTube clip offers an explanation of how this works.

4. Division

Division is the process of splitting or separating a number into equal parts. It is really important that you look at how the nursing problem is phrased so you are clear about which number is the divisor (the number doing the dividing) and which is the dividend (the number being divided). This is where nurses often make errors in their calculations. With division you move from left to right to find an answer so start with the largest number and work towards the smallest.

- **Division using traditional method**

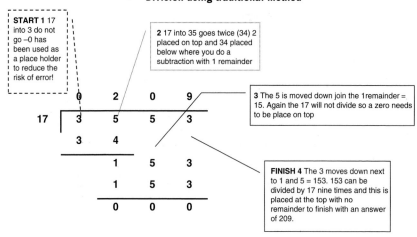

START 1 17 into 3 do not go –0 has been used as a place holder to reduce the risk of error!

2 17 into 35 goes twice (34) 2 placed on top and 34 placed below where you do a subtraction with 1 remainder

3 The 5 is moved down join the 1 remainder = 15. Again the 17 will not divide so a zero needs to be place on top

FINISH 4 The 3 moves down next to 1 and 5 = 153. 153 can be divided by 17 nine times and this is placed at the top with no remainder to finish with an answer of 209.

The final answer: 3553 divided by 17 = 209

When working with numbers that are not easy to divide it is worth using a separate multiplication lattice as below:

$17 \times 1 = 17$
$17 \times 2 = 34$
$17 \times 3 = 51$
$17 \times 4 = 68$
$17 \times 5 = 85$
$17 \times 6 = 101$
$17 \times 7 = 119$
$17 \times 8 = 136$
$17 \times 9 = 153$

The zero is included during the calculation stage though it does not need to be there, that is, the final answer is 209. It is there as a place holder to prevent errors happening during the calculation stage. It is also very easy to forget the 0 that is in the middle by ignoring it and again this will result in a serious computation error.

- **Division using space-saving method**

	0	2	0	9
17	3	³5	¹5	¹⁵3

Rather than placing the numbers underneath in rows as in the previous method the numbers and remainders are moved along the sum, that is, what is left over as a remainder is passed along to the neighbour, like passing a baton in a relay. So 17 does not go into 3 so the 3 moves next to the 5 to make 35. 17 fits in twice – 2 moves to the top and the remainder of 1 passes to the neighbour to make 15 and so on! Ensure that you do not ignore the '0' that appears between the 2 and the 9. Errors may occur here when the 0 is ignored or not recorded.

Improving your maths vocabulary – Factors are numbers that will divide exactly into another number without leaving a remainder.

It is worth looking at the numbers to see how easy it is going to be to divide them in terms of factorisation. For example, a number is divisible by 2 if the final digit is a multiple of 2 (e.g. 0, 2, 4 etc.). For example, 184, 2098 and 380. A number is divisible by 3 if the sum of the digits is a multiple of 3 (e.g. 3, 6, 9 etc.). For example, 573, 903, and 39 (5 + 7 + 3 = 15, 9 + 0 + 3 = 12 and 3 + 9 = 12). A number is divisible by 5 if the final digit is either 0 or 5. For example, 80, 3665 and 380.

There are many other tests for divisibility, but in terms of keeping things simple these are the most useful to look for. Have a look at the online activity and test the theory by looking to see which numbers are divisible by 2, 3 and 5. This is really useful when using formulae and simplifying fractions (see Chapter 4) so as to simplify the mathematical processes you are undertaking, particularly when not using a calculator.

Words used to define 'division'	Symbols
Divide, Division, Quotient, Goes Into, How Many Times, factors	**÷ or /**

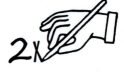

Dividing numbers (round to two decimal places)

- $94 \div 6 =$
- $194 \div 26 =$
- $1073 \div 11 =$
- $10.1 \div 3.2 =$
- $8.99 \div 7.4 =$

As already discussed there are rules that apply to certain operations. One way of remembering which order to do the steps when formulae are introduced is the following:

BoDMAS or BiDMAS

The order of operations **B**rackets, power **O**f or **I**ndices to cover the O or I, then **D**ivision, **M**ultiplication, **A**ddition and **S**ubtraction.

This means that if you are presented with a calculation you need to first complete the sum in the brackets and then complete them in the order above.

Some addition, subtraction, multiplication and division jokes to amuse you and/or to use to entertain young children (answers at the end of the book)

A poem about mathematics

A boy was teaching girl arithmetic, he said, it was his mission.

He kissed her once; he kissed her twice and said, 'now that's addition'.

In silent satisfaction, she sweetly gave him kisses back and said 'now that's subtraction'.

Then he kissed her, she kissed him, without an explanation.

And both together smiled and said 'that's multiplication'.

Then her dad appeared upon the scene and made a quick decision,

He kicked the boy three streets away and said 'that's long division!'

Can you work out the answers?
- Why was the snake so good at numeracy?
- What tools do you need for numeracy?
- Why is arithmetic hard work?

APPLYING BASIC NUMERICAL OPERATIONS TO THE NURSING OF CHILDREN AND YOUNG PEOPLE

Fluid balance – the theory

Monitoring fluid balance is an essential requirement in nursing practice, whether nursing infant, child or young person. A common healthcare example that uses addition and subtraction involves calculating the fluid balance of a patient. Fluid balance is a simple but very useful way to estimate whether a patient is either becoming dehydrated or overloaded with liquids. It is calculated, on a daily basis, by adding up the total volume of liquid that has gone into their body (drinks, oral liquid medicines, intravenous drips, transfusions), then adding up the total volume of liquid that has come out of their body (urine, wound drains, blood lost during surgery, vomit). The fluid balance is then calculated by subtracting the total output from the total input, and is generally quoted in millilitres. You record this by using a fluid balance (or input–output) chart.

So let us use the case scenario to explore the numbers that relate to Tommy by exploring why fluid balance is so important and how to analyse the data we are presented with by observing Tommy, measuring vital signs and looking at laboratory results.

Water forms 45–75% of total body weight. An infant has the highest amount of water per body weight, that is, premature infant at 90%, newborn infant at 70–80% and at 1–2 years 64%. Homeostasis of the human body relies on fluid, electrolyte and acid–base balance, where you need balance between four fluids: intracellular fluid (ICF), intravascular fluid (IVF), interstitial fluid (ISF) and extracellular fluid (ECF).

Movement between the vascular space and tissues depends on osmotic pressure or force, oncotic pressure, hydrostatic pressure and capillary permeability. Solutes within the compartments of the body (intracellular (IC), extracellular (EC), which is subdivided down further into interstitial, intravascular and transcellular fluid) move through the membranes separating those compartments. The membranes are semi-permeable allowing some solutes to pass through but not others. Solutes move through membranes at cellular level by diffusion, active transport osmosis. These solutes include sodium and glucose which move readily across capillary membrane. Plasma proteins maintain effective osmolality by generating plasma oncotic pressure (the ability of plasma proteins to hold water). Sodium is most abundant in the ECF and is responsible for the osmotic balance of this space. Potassium maintains osmotic balance within ICF. ICF maintains a fairly steady osmotic balance, where the aim is to maintain osmotic equilibrium. Infants have a higher proportion of ECF compared to older children and adults so as a result are more at risk of developing dehydration because ECF is more easily lost from the body than ICF (Willcock and Jewkes, 2000).

At its most basic children have a higher metabolic rate and a greater body surface area which means that turnover of fluid is faster and any, even minor, disturbance will cause problems with hydration more rapidly than for adults. As a result, as with the situation with Tommy, who has gastroenteritis, deterioration in the form of dehydration, potentially progressing to shock, could happen very quickly. Gastroenteritis in children, characterised by sudden onset of diarrhoea, which can be with or without vomiting, is most commonly caused by an enteric virus though it can have bacterial or protozoal causes (NICE, 2009). The aim for Tommy is to assess his level of hydration and start treatment to rehydrate as quickly as possible thus preventing the potential risk of hypovolaemic shock.

Positive and negative balances

The body maintains a dynamic balance between fluid intake and output – the process for making these final adjustments to achieve this balance is called homeostasis. Ideally, the total volume of fluid that goes into a child should balance the total volume that eventually comes out of them, so the difference in the total input and output should be almost zero. However, if the fluid balance is positive, then this indicates that more fluid is going in than is coming out (i.e. there is more fluid on-board which is not necessarily a bad thing if, for instance, they were admitted suffering from dehydration as is the subject of this chapter, Tommy). A negative fluid balance indicates that more fluid is coming out than is going in and the child is at risk of becoming dehydrated, though clearly you cannot look at the fluid balance in isolation from other signs and symptoms. As with the monitoring of vital signs in the previous chapter you have to look at the big picture using all numerical measures and observations.

Insensible loss

Insensible loss mostly occurs through the skin and respiratory tract and can be calculated at 30 mL/kg/24 hr. Fever will increase insensible loss by 12% per 1°C rise in temperature above 37.2°C. This will have an impact on Tommy who has a raised temperature. Fluid lost from the body in perspiration and breathing is proportional to body surface area, which is approximately 300 mL/m²/day and can be calculated using the following formula, which we used in the previous chapter to calculate body surface area.

$$BSA = \sqrt{\frac{Weight \times Height}{3600}}$$

$$Insensible\ fluid\ loss = 300 \times BSA$$

Source: Willcock and Jewkes (2000)

A new symbol appears in this calculation. This is nothing to worry about as we add a new symbol to our collection. Calculating square roots involves a number multiplied by itself to give an answer so, for example, the square root of $16 = 4$, that is, $(4 \times 4 = 16)$.

It is quite difficult to calculate a square number unless it is a perfect square so this is where a calculator would be needed though again you can estimate to the nearest whole number to check the answer that the calculator will give you.

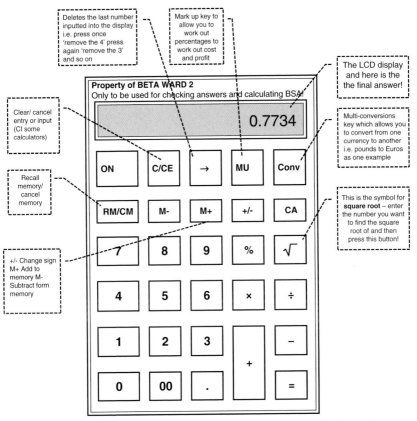

Deletes the last number inputted into the display i.e. press once 'remove the 4' press again 'remove the 3' and so on

Mark up key to allow you to work out percentages to work out cost and profit

The LCD display and here is the the final answer!

Clear/ cancel entry or input (CI some calculators)

Property of BETA WARD 2
Only to be used for checking answers and calculating BSA!

0.7734

Multi-conversions key which allows you to convert from one currency to another i.e. pounds to Euros as one example

Recall memory/ cancel memory

This is the symbol for **square root** – enter the number you want to find the square root of and then press this button!

+/- Change sign M+ Add to memory M- Subtract form memory

ON	C/CE	→	MU	Conv
RM/CM	M-	M+	+/-	CA
7	8	9	%	√
4	5	6	×	÷
1	2	3		−
0	00	.	+	=

Understanding your calculator – you probably know how to use your calculator in the most basic way – this diagram allows you to explore it further and find out what some of the buttons you do not use mean!

The calculator diagram identifies the square root key and some of the functions of other keys on a basic calculator. As with any other piece of equipment (see Chapter 2) you should be able to use a calculator with confidence. Please note that not all the keys on all calculators have the same names and functions, though obviously the core symbols are the same!

Do you remember the games you used to play on your calculator at school? Turn the book upside down and have a look at the diagram of the calculator – what is it saying to

you? Using your pocket calculator is another way to distract and use play with older children and young people.

Here is how you get to the word in a roundabout way, which will allow you to play with your calculator:

Enter 6.2, multiply by itself, then add 0.23, divide by 50 then turn calculator upside down and you have a result!

Visit the website Section 4 for links to some maths games and puzzles using a calculator.

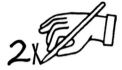

Calculate Tommy's insensible loss.

Worked example: Calculating fluid balance on Day 1 of Tommy's admission

For ease of calculation we can use the following approximations though these will obviously vary dependent on clinical state on admission, that is, the factors related to Tommy are:

On Day 1 of his admission, over 24 hours, Tommy receives 845 mL intravenously and has drunk 300 mL of ORS. He has vomited 350 mL, passed 600 mL of urine and also had five bouts of diarrhoea (not measured).

The fluid balance is the difference between the total fluid input and the total fluid output during a day. The first thing we need to do is ensure that we are using the metric unit of millilitres (and not fluid ounces).

Then add together all the fluid inputs in millilitres, that is, 845 mL + 300 mL = 1145 mL.

Then add together all the fluid outputs in millilitres, that is, 350 mL + 600 mL = 950 mL.

The fluid balance is the daily total inputs minus the daily total outputs, that is, 1145 − 950 = 195 mL.

This is a positive fluid balance, indicating that Tommy is taking on more fluid than he is losing. If the output had been larger than the input, then the fluid balance would be a negative number (e.g. input 2000 mL – output 2500 mL = –500 mL fluid balance). The reason for this is because Tommy is dehydrated and clearly needs to take on more fluid rather than less and we have also not been able to manage to measure his outputs accurately so this is not 100% accurate.

We have also not taken account of his insensible loss which needs to be added to output, that is, 165 mL, that is, 950 mL + 165 mL = 1115 mL which then means that his is a positive balance of 30 mL – all but in balance in effect.

There is a Day 2 fluid balance chart for you to look at and work out if Tommy is in a positive or negative balance.

The most accurate way of assessing Tommy's hydration state is to weigh him first thing in the morning and compare it with admission weight and/or most recent weight if known.

1 mL = 1 mg (though please note that this rule applies to water only, which is why we can only use it as a guide for healthcare practice when measuring input and output).

What are negative numbers?

We have already briefly considered negative numbers in the previous chapter when discussing temperature, though this needs to be more explicitly defined.

Negative numbers are used to represent loss or absence, because the numbers in effect are less than zero, that is, a debt or scales that fall below zero (as in temperature) or below the bottom line and, in this context, the balance between fluid intake and output.

Symbols used to represent these numbers – positive (+) and negative (−).

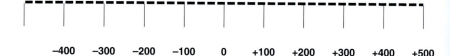

−400	−300	−200	−100	0	+100	+200	+300	+400	+500

Using number lines can help you work out positive and negative amounts when adding them up as shown above in the worked example.

Skills and competences in relation to managing hydration in children and young people

- **Assessing hydration**

Defining the terms

Sodium is key to managing fluid balance as well as water. They have a close relationship where sodium attracts water – osmotic pull. A reduction in sodium within the tissues will result in less osmotic pull and less water will move to tissue fluids. Sodium is a positively charged cation and has many functions including fluid balance, muscle function, acid–base balance and maintaining electrical balance (ALSG, 2011).

- Isotonic dehydration exists when sodium and water are lost proportionately (serum sodium 130–150 mmol/L).
- Hyponatraemic dehydration exists when a greater proportion of sodium is lost (serum sodium is less than 130 mmol/L). This can be caused by sodium loss from gastrointestinal tract due to aspiration, vomiting, diarrhoea or paralytic ileus.
- Hypernatraemic dehydration exists when a greater proportion of water is lost (serum sodium is greater than 150 mmol/ L). This can happen due to reduced fluid intake, diarrhoea, vomiting and polyuria.

Normal values of sodium.

Age range	Normal values
Adult	135–146 mmol/L
Child	136–143 mmol/L
Neonate	133–146 mmol/L

Source: Skinner (2005)

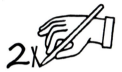

From the information offered at the beginning of this chapter what type of dehydration is Tommy exhibiting?

NPSA alert 22 (2007c)

The common practice of giving children 4% dextrose and 0.18% sodium chloride (called 4¹/₅ for short) was stopped following an NPSA alert identifying the risks associated with this fluid and hospital-acquired hyponatraemia. The recommendation was to replace this hypotonic solution with one with a higher percentage of sodium chloride, that is, 0.45% sodium chloride and 5% glucose (hypotonic) or if a child is at high risk of developing hyponatraemia, that is, peri- or post-operatively sodium chloride 0.9% with glucose 5% (isotonic). This needs to be decided on an individual basis for each child depending on the clinical presentation.

- **Estimating weight**

The previous chapter outlines the process for estimating weight and we will use the following information to calculate Tommy's weight:

0–12 months	(0.5 × age in months) + 4
1–5 years	(2 × age in years) + 8
6–12 years	(3 × age in years) + 7

Source: ILCOR 2010 (APLS version 5.0) resuscitation guidelines

These guidelines have been updated and you can see the difference from the way we used to estimate children's weights, that is, using Age + 4 × 2, that is, 4 kg difference which will have an impact when calculating fluids and drug dosages in an emergency situation.

There are more examples on the online resource so you can practise estimating weight for the other children who are case study examples in this text book.

Unless we have the recent weight for Tommy we will not be able to base our assessment of level of dehydration based on weight, so we have used clinical signs taking account of the fact that this is not an exact science.

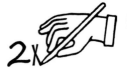

What is Tommy's estimated weight?

- **Capillary refill time**

As already discussed in the previous chapter, how to do it? Press with a finger on the child's forehead or sternum for 5 seconds then release. When the pressure is released colour returns to the area within 2 seconds. A slower refill time than this indicates poor skin perfusion which may be due to hypovolaemia (in this case caused by dehydration).

- **Calculating fluid requirements**

The method for calculating fluid requirements is as follows:

4 mL/kg/hr for the first 10 kg of body weight or
     100 mL/kg/day
2 mL/kg/hr for the second 10 kg body weight or
     50 mL/kg/day
1 mL/kg/hr for each additional kg body weight or
     20 mL/kg/day

Example:

A 12 kg child would require 1000 (first 10 kg) + 100 (2 kg) = 1100 mL/day

A 27 kg child would require 1000 (first 10 kg 17 kg remain) + 500 (second 10 kg – 7 kg remain) + 140 (last 7 kg no remainder) = 1640 mL

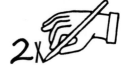

Tommy weighs 11.8 kg, so what are his daily fluid requirements?

Calculating fluid deficit

A child's fluid can be calculated following an estimation of the degree of dehydration expressed as percentage of body weight. (e.g. a 10 kg child who is 5% dehydrated has a water deficit of 500 mL). The deficit is replaced over a time period that varies according to the child's condition, taking account of the fact that this is an inexact science where estimation as a skill in numeracy is vital. The rate of rehydration should be individualised and adjusted with ongoing assessment of the child.

% Dehydration × Weight (kg) × 10 = Weight in grams = Amount deficit in millilitre

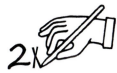

Tommy is assessed as 5% dehydrated (mild), so what extra fluids will he need to correct this deficit?

How to estimate the percentage dehydration?

Clinical sign	Mild (5% or 50 mL/kg)	Moderate (10% or 100 mL/kg)	Severe (>15% or>150 mL/kg)
Capillary refill	1–2 seconds (normal)	>2 seconds (normal to delayed)	>3 seconds (prolonged)
Mucous membranes	Normal	Dry	Parched, cracked
Skin turgor	Normal	Mild, reduced	Decreased
Respirations	Normal	Increased	Deep acidotic breathing
Urine output	Decreased	Oliguria	Oligura/anuria

Note: This is the chart used at Arch Mede Hospital.

Initially Tommy starts on a regime of Oral Rehydration therapy using an oral rehydration solution (ORS) then, due to continued vomiting, was commenced on intravenous fluids as per NICE (2009) guidelines.

Management of mild dehydration

Children without clinical manifestations of dehydration are usually managed by encouraging fluid intake, discouraging fruit juices and carbonated drinks and offering ORS as supplemental if at risk of becoming dehydrated. Children who are mildly dehydrated should again be managed with

ORS at 50 mL/kg for fluid deficit over 4 hours as well as maintenance fluid given frequently and in small amounts and can be given via a nasogastric tube if they are unable to drink or if vomiting. The move to intravenous fluids will be considered if they show red flag symptoms and signs such as signs of deterioration, altered responsiveness, sunken eyes and tachypnoea or tachycardia or if there is no improvement with ORS therapy and the child is vomiting (NICE, 2009).

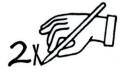

What was the total amount of ORS that Tommy needed to drink to overcome his fluid deficit? (The answer should be the same as the one calculated above – can you see why?)

Calculating flow rates

In children's nursing practice we use electronic devices to control flow rate of fluids so we do not often have to calculate drip rates. However you should still be able to do this so this section will consider how to calculate hourly rates of fluids and also drip rate calculations.

To calculate an hourly rate all you need to do is divide the total maintenance fluids to be administered over the time they need to be administered, that is, for Tommy this will be 1090 (total daily fluids) divided by 24 = 45.42 mL/hr

To calculate the drip rate (drops per millilitre of solution (drops/mL)) you need to know the drop factor of the giving set, which will be written on the packaging. For most standard giving sets this is 20 drops/mL. For giving sets for blood administration it is usually 15 drops/mL.

Method 1

Using a formula

$$\frac{\text{Total IV fluid (in mL)}}{\text{Total minutes}} \times \frac{\text{Drop factor}}{1} = \frac{\text{Drip rate}}{\text{(drops/min)}}$$

For Tommy:

$$\frac{1090}{1440} \times \frac{20}{1} = \textbf{15.2 drops/min}$$

Method 2

Calculate how much fluid needs to be administered intravenously per hour = 45.42 mL (as worked out above)

Then divide by 60 to get the rate per minute = 0.76 mL/min

Now multiply by the drop rate per minute = 0.76 × 20 = 15.2 drops/min

Note: Please note that there is no rounding up done during this calculation – can only do this at the end where you would round up to 15 drops/min, though for a child of Tommy's age this will be administered via an electronic device.

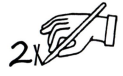

Have a go at the following examples:

- 1 unit of blood (450 mL) is administered over 4 hours. What will be the hourly rate and the drop rate?
- 1½ L of sodium chloride 0.9% with glucose 5% over 12 hours. What will be the hourly rate and the drop rate?

Remember that to maintain adequate hydration (and not overhydrate) you need to take account of other inputs. This is particularly important for neonates where you may need to make adjustments to the maintenance fluids to take account of other inputs, that is, medications, feeds etc. In Tommy's case as he started to tolerate oral fluids and stopped vomiting the fluid rate was reduced accordingly and stopped at the beginning of Day 3.

Dependent on reason for admission you may also want to administer a certain percentage of the total maintenance fluids, that is, for children who have suffered head trauma you may restrict fluids to reduce the risk of raised intracranial pressure and cerebral oedema so you may give 60% of the total maintenance. We will look at how to calculate this in the next chapter.

OUTCOMES IN RELATION TO TOMMY

You will want to know how Tommy got on during his hospital stay. It took 3 days to correct his dehydration and he was unable to tolerate the ORS, due to continuing vomiting, so was rehydrated using an intravenous infusion and discharged home once tolerating diet and fluids. He was diagnosed with a viral infection, Rotavirus, whose symptoms include watery diarrhoea, fever, vomiting and respiratory symptoms and is very common in children particularly during the winter months. Needless to say his siblings and other children at his nursery were also unwell though Mrs Turing was able to manage the illness at home by giving frequent small amounts of ORS.

CONCLUDING COMMENTS

This chapter has covered the numeracy skills of addition, subtraction, multiplication and division in some detail and set the skills within the context of monitoring fluid balance with a 2-year-old child.

At this stage it is worth reflecting on progress and making some decision with regard to the best methods of calculation that work for you particularly for long multiplication and long division. You will also have had an opportunity to practise some weight and fluid calculation as well as managing positive and negative balances and numbers.

Whilst the focus of this chapter has been on the basic skills of adding, subtracting, multiplying and dividing we have started to move off into the world of parts of number by looking at percentages which will now be considered in much greater depth and detail in the next chapter.

Chapter 4

ADVANCING ONWARDS: TAKING THE WHOLE NUMBER APART

Numeracy in Children's Nursing, First Edition. Arija Parker
© 2015 John Wiley & Sons, Ltd. Published 2015 by John Wiley & Sons Ltd.

LEARNING FOCUS

From Whole Number to Part of a Number
The focus of this chapter will be to look at part of a number in the form of fractions, percentages (including decimals), ratio and proportion and why these numerical skills are needed and how they are applied to the nursing of children and young people.

LEARNING OUTCOMES

By the end of this chapter you should be able to:

- Calculate using fractions, percentages, ratios and proportion
- Apply these, and other numerical skills, to common scenarios in children and young people's nursing practice
- Round up decimal numbers to the correct (or requested) number of places
- Add to your general knowledge about the nutritional needs of children and young people using BMI formula, growth charts and other useful tools and information sources

CASE SCENARIO 4

Edward Euler (5 months) has been admitted to a cubicle on Beta Ward 2 (The Children's Unit) as a referral from his health visitor, because she is worried about his weight gain – he appears to be failing to thrive. Edward was born at full term weighing 3.5 kg. His present weight, on admission to the ward, is 6.3 kg. He is accompanied by his mother, Melanie Euler. She is living with her partner of 2 years (Edward's dad), who is at work at the time of admission. He has three siblings, Ellie (2), Eugenie (4) and Esther (6). Melanie breastfed Edward until he was 4 months, when she returned to part-time work as a teaching assistant. He is now on infant formula milk and she has started weaning diet, even though she has been advised by her health visitor that the WHO/DH guidance is that weaning should only start at 6 months. She is worried about Edward's poor growth and development and the fact that he appears to be hungry all the time.

The clinical issues discussed in this chapter will focus on dietary intake, how to calculate requirements for the under 1s and also cover some of the investigations undertaken to find out why Edward is failing to thrive.

Children who are failing to thrive are diagnosed on the basis that their weight is lower than the third percentile or 20% below the ideal weight for height (see his growth chart in Section 1).

Hospital number	AMH2014-04
Ward number	Beta Ward 2 (The children's unit)

Temperature	Pulse	Blood pressure	Respirations	CRT	Pain score	PEWS
37.5°C	140 bpm	Not recorded on admission	38 breaths per minute	2 seconds	0	0

As a starter activity have a look at the numerical information offered and start having a think about what might be happening to Edward by having a practice at the activities below.

As discussed in Chapter 2, by the age of 5 months, Edward should have doubled his birth weight so what should his weight be?

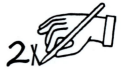

Feed calculation for Edward
The first task on admission is to work out Edward's feed requirements to ensure that he is meeting his nutritional requirements thus utilising skills developed from Chapter 3 – that is, multiplication and addition skills. Calculate Edward's requirements based on his actual weight and estimated weight using the information in the table below.

Age of infant	Total fluid in 24 hours (mL/kg)
Newborn	30
2 days	60
3 days	90
4 days	120
5 days	150
1 week to 8 months	150
9–12 months	120

CASE SCENARIO 5

Nathan (9) has been admitted to Gamma Ward 3 (The Children's Day Case Surgery Unit) for dental extractions under general anaesthetic (GA). He is accompanied by his father, Mr. Newton, who is very anxious about the admission, because at preoperative assessment there were concerns raised about Nathan's weight and, as a result, suitability for surgery and GA. He lives with his mum and dad and is the only child of the Newton family. Mum is very obese and housebound, which is why dad, who has taken a day off work, is accompanying Nathan to hospital. Dad has a body mass index (BMI) in the normal range for his height and weight. The focus for this chapter will be around the numbers that relate to Nathan's obesity, in terms of BMI and growth, as well as some nutritional information to aid weight management. He is having dental extractions due to dental caries, caused by poor dental hygiene and a high carbohydrate diet – Nathan has a very sweet tooth! His birth weight was 4.1 kg and his weight on admission is 42.5 kg (height 131 cm) and he is aged 9 years and 8 months on admission.

Hospital number	AMH2014–05
Ward number	Gamma Ward 3 (The Children's Day Case Surgery Unit)

Temperature	Pulse	Blood pressure	Respirations	CRT	Pain score	PEWS
36.9°C	90 bpm	120/80	26 breaths per minute	2 seconds	2	0

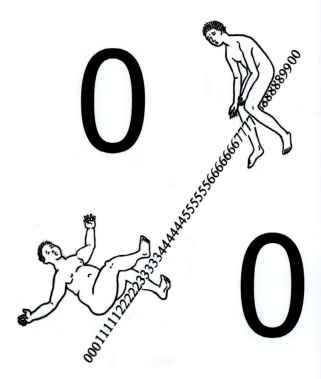

INTRODUCTION

This chapter will explore the world of parts of a whole number and so will focus in on the use of fractions and percentages in nursing and healthcare practice as well as explore the use of ratio and proportion as other methods for calculation in children's nursing practice. Examples from Edward and Nathan's experiences as well as other relevant aspects of nursing practice will be utilised to ensure that contextual relevance to numeracy is present throughout.

Setting the context

The NMC (2010) in their standards for Pre-registration Nursing Education ESC 27 states that newly registered graduate nurses should be able to assist patients (including children and young people) to choose a diet that provides an adequate nutritional and fluid intake and

'Accurately monitors dietary and fluid intake and completes relevant documentation' (NMC, 2010, p. 129)

and from ESC 28:

'Takes and records accurate measurements of weight, height, length, BMI and other appropriate measures of nutritional status' and at entry to register 'Makes a comprehensive assessment of people's needs in relation to nutrition identifying, documenting and communicating level of risk' (NMC, 2010, p. 130).

These are the competences that apply and will be explored in relation to the numeracy skills under discussion in this chapter. We will also consider how to create an environment that is conducive to eating and drinking (ESC 30, NMC, 2012), as well as offering health promotion advice, from the perspective of the two children who are the focus of numeracy activity in this chapter.

FRACTIONS

At its most simplest a fraction can be defined as a part of one.

The illustrated maths dictionary definition (2006) is: A number written where the bottom part (denominator) tells you how many parts that one or the whole is divided into and the top part (numerator) tells you how many parts you have. If the numerator and denominator are the same the fraction equals 1.

Tucker (2001) states the fact that many students fall off the ladder of mathematical learning when they encounter fractions. This will tend to happen at the primary school stage of education so many nursing students enter the profession without understanding fractions. The aim of this section is to demystify the process and identify how useful they can be in nursing numeracy practice.

To return to earlier chapters, when discussing fractions, the critical concept to consider is the units, which is a standard reference for measurement or counting. Tucker (2001) defines the units as a standard which can vary from centimetres to degrees to amounts in cups, when either baking or explaining how much a patient needs to drink in a day. When using the imperial system it was vital to understand how fractions relate to each other as units, that is, when you look a ruler which has inches on it you will see that it is split into halves, fourths, eighths. We do need to think about units and measurement where time is included in our calculations, that is, ½ an hour is equal to 30 minutes.

Fractions are best understood in diagrammatic format though rather than using the traditional pizza used in school education. Let us use lots of different shapes as well as the Eatwell plate (see later) to illustrate the point.

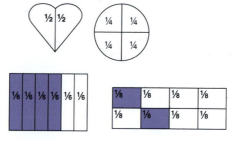

This is the most common way of demonstrating how fractions work though please remember that each piece needs to be equal to form an equal fraction, that is, you cannot just split, for example, the circle into three random sized pieces for each piece to equal a 1/3.

So you can see straight away from this simple example that there are relationships between fractions – called **equivalent fractions**, which means that we can cancel down and simplify fractions to make them easier to work with. This is an important concept to understand before we look at nursing formulae, which also allows you to see why we do not necessarily need to use a formula to calculate in children's nursing practice. For example, 4/8 (four-eights) is the same as a ½ and 2/6 (two-sixths) is the same as ⅓. If we think about common children's nursing calculations where we may require 60 mg of paracetamol where it is supplied as 120 mg = 1 teaspoonful (5 mL) the fraction we need will be 60/120 which can be simplified to ½ so we will give half a teaspoonful (or 2.5 mL).

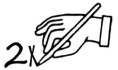

2x

Have a closer look at the figures above and identify what fraction of the area is shaded in its simplified form?

If we look closely at equivalent fractions, that is, fractions that can be cancelled down to simpler units, both numbers usually end with a 0, 5 or an even number where nursing calculations are involved. So any number that ends with a zero can be divided by 10, 5 or 2 which is very useful to know when looking at nursing calculations where these numbers abound.

Fractions that have numbers which cannot be cancelled down or simplified are called vulgar fractions, that is, 5/6ths, 9/10ths. Returning to the content of Chapter 1 you can see that these numbers are prime and odd numbers which partially explains why we cannot simplify them. They result in recurring decimals where there is a pattern of numbers which continue to infinity, that is, 1/3 = 0.33333333. Why are they called vulgar? The term comes from the Latin meaning 'common people' and they are sometimes referred to as common fractions or simple fractions and include all fractions where there is a number above a line and below a line neither of which is a zero – the most commonly occurring fractions.

Fractions where the top number (numerator) is bigger than the bottom number (denominator) are called improper fractions, that is, 9/4 – 9 quarters, 11/8 – 11 eighths. These may also be called mixed number fractions, though written as 2¼, 1⅜ in relation to the previous examples. So the converse is true – a fraction which is less than a whole unit and numerator that is smaller than the denominator is a proper fraction.

Remember whatever you do to the top number (numerator) you must do the same to the bottom (denominator) and you need to go one step at a time if you plan to do multiple operations.

There are many worksheets and links to websites that will allow you to practice working with fractions (see Section 2 and Activity 4 A).

Whilst we do not necessarily need to be able to do the following fraction sums, to aid comprehension it is useful to carry on experimenting with fractions and learn how to do the following. This will then allow you to understand how and why we use nursing formulae.

Adding and subtracting fractions

The key is ensuring that the bottom number (denominator) is the same in both fractions that are being added together or subtracted from each other. You just need to leave the denominator the same and add the numerators together as shown below.

$$\frac{2}{8} + \frac{3}{8} = \frac{5}{8}$$

$$\frac{5}{6} - \frac{4}{6} = \frac{1}{6}$$

If the denominator is not the same we have to find a way of making them the same by equalising them, that is, by multiplying the two denominators together you will be able to get a common denominator of 30. You then need to multiply the numerators 5 by 5 to get 25 and 4 by 6 to get 24.

$$\frac{5}{6} - \frac{4}{5} = \frac{25 - 24}{30} = \frac{1}{30}$$

Multiplying and dividing fractions

This activity is important because we routinely multiply fractions when using nursing formulae. Learning to cancel down and cross-cancel (as already mentioned earlier on) is a very useful skill to have to simplify the numeracy operations, which we sometimes omit to do thus leading us to work with very complex numbers unnecessarily.

This is easy in comparison with adding and subtracting whereby you multiply numerators and denominators separately.

Example with simple fraction.

$$\frac{3}{7} \times \frac{4}{5} = \frac{12}{35}$$

Example with cancelling down.

$$\frac{15 \ (\div 5 = 3)}{35 \ (\div 5 = 7)} \times \frac{20 \ (\div 5 = 4)}{25 \ (\div 5 = 5)} = \frac{12}{35}$$

Can you see that the numbers can be cancelled down by dividing top and bottom by 5 in the first fraction and by 5 in the second or you could cross-cancel the 15 and 25 and the 20 and 25 by dividing by 5 to get exactly the same result?

Dividing involves turning the second fraction upside down, that is, if you want to divide ¾ by 1/3 it will look like this in the final division which happens then to turn into a multiplication.

$$\frac{3}{4} \times \frac{3}{1} = \frac{9}{4}$$

If this does not make sense to you remember the following:

'Ours is not to reason why, just invert and multiply'

Though you can think about a simple division, that is, dividing ½ by ½ is obviously 1, that is, ½ ÷ ½ = ½ × 2/1 = 2/2 = 1.

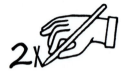

Who invented fractions?

REVISITING DECIMAL NUMBERS

How do you turn a fraction into a decimal?

This is very easy because you just divide top (numerator) by bottom (denominator), that is, ½ = 1 divided by 2 = 0.5, 2/5 = 2 divided by 5 = 0.4.

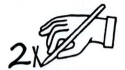

Have a go at the following examples:

5/8, 15/40, 5/6, 7/9, 28/96

You will notice that you have got numbers that go on to infinity as a result of some of these examples. There is a new symbol to add in this instance whereby for numbers that repeat themselves, that is, 1/3 = 0.333…. you add a dot on the first and last repeating pattern in this case over the 3, that is, 0.3̇. If the pattern was 6.125125125.... you would add dots over the 1 and 5, that is, 6.1̇25̇ This also takes us neatly on to a discussion around when to round and when not to round...... that is the question.

Rounding decimals

When you turn a fraction into a decimal you will often end up with numerous numbers after the decimal point. On numeracy tests you will be asked to round to a certain number of decimal places.

That is, 7.345 rounded to two decimal places would be 7.35. To work out how to do this look at the number in the third (or final) decimal place which allows you to make the decision around whether you round up or leave the second decimal place number the same. If it is 5 or above it goes up – if it is below 5 it stays the same.

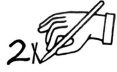

- 175.33333 (round to one decimal place)
- 7.7689 (round to two decimal places)
- 125.9534 (round to three decimal places)

Most usually we would do this when calculating infusion rates though it has to be remembered that when rounding dosages prescribed on a prescription chart a small amount of rounding up or down could make a massive difference to the amount a young child or neonate receives so doses should be prescribed accurately (with consideration to the form it is to be given in) thus avoiding the potential for error.

Examples of fractions in nursing practice

At this point we can introduce the Eatwell plate which illustrates the numeracy concepts under discussion, that is, fractions, percentages and proportions of the main food groups in relation to each other. Does this help explain this to children and young people or do you think it is self-explanatory?

The eatwell plate

Use the eatwell plate to help you get the balance right. It shows how much of what you eat should come from each food group.

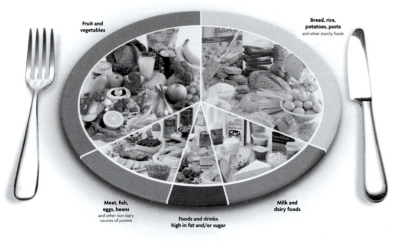

Department of Health in association with the Welsh Assembly Government, the Scottish Government and the Food Standards Agency in Northern Ireland

The Eatwell plate; another way of recording this information could be in a table as below.

Green	Yellow	Blue	Purple	Pink
Fruit and vegetables	Bread, rice, potatoes, pasta and other starchy food	Milk and dairy products i.e. cheese, yoghurts	Food and drinks high in fat and/or sugar	Meat, fish, eggs, beans and other non-dairy sources of protein
33%	33%	15%	8%	12%
⅓	⅓	3/20	2/25	3/25

The table is constructed to scale so that Nathan and his dad can see how much food should be eaten from each food group approximately, though from this starting point they now need to know how much of each group can be eaten on a daily basis to be healthy.

Portion sizes

What size is a portion of fruit in the 5 A DAY approach to ensuring you eat enough fruit and vegetables every day?

NHS 5 A DAY website
http://www.nhs.uk/LiveWell/5ADAY/Pages/5ADAYhome.aspx

Change for life

http://www.nhs.uk/Change4Life/Pages/five-a-day.aspx

This will also give you some links and materials to give to Nathan and his dad as they start to think about what they eat and what they could change to help Nathan and his mum to lose weight. One thing that Nathan asks is what 5 A DAY actually means and asks if 5 grapes will do?

Nathan has identified some foods that he likes and these are included in the table below to indicate what is equivalent to an adult portion size. This should help you give advice with regard to what constitutes a portion as well as what counts for your 5 A DAY, though think about how you will explain this both to Nathan and his dad.

Food	Adult portion size for this food group	Amount	Additional notes
Bananas	Fruit = 80 g	I medium banana	These are the only fruits Nathan will eat
Grapes		1 handful	
Fruit juice		150 mL	Juices only count as 1 of your 5 A DAY however much you drink.
Raisins	Dried fruit = 30 g	1 tablespoon	Nathan will have a small box of these as part of his packed lunch.

(continued)

Food	Adult portion size for this food group	Amount	Additional notes
Potatoes	Vegetables = 80 g	Do not count as part of 5 A DAY	Nathan loves potatoes in any shape or form especially chips. Unfortunately they do not count towards your 5 A DAY, because of their classification a starchy (carbohydrate) food, and used in place of other sources of starch such as bread, rice or pasta.
Kidney beans		3 heaped tablespoons	Nathan will eat these if part of a chilli con carne if chopped up and disguised in the food. Beans and pulses count as a maximum of one portion a day, however much you eat. This is because, while pulses contain fibre, they do not give the same mixture of vitamins, minerals and other nutrients as fruit and vegetables.
Carrots		3 heaped tablespoons	Nathan will eat these cooked
Peas (frozen)		3 heaped tablespoons	Nathan loves peas.

Source: NHS Choices – 5 A DAY Portion sizes, accessed at:http://www.nhs.uk/Livewell/5ADAY/Documents/Downloads/5ADAY_portion_guide.pdf

The Change 4 life campaign is another great resource for Nathan to explore issues of healthiness in a simple and fun way, which is similar to many health-related campaigns in other countries, by focusing in on 'me sized meals', though again this does not clearly identify what a portion size for a child is, though the guidance is to compare fist sizes and use handful sizes and cups/mugs to estimate portion sizes.

This link takes you to the website so that you can find out more! Change 4 life:
http://www.nhs.uk/Change4Life/Pages/kids-portion-sizes.aspx

The language of fractions

In the same way that we looked at the language of operations such as addition and subtraction in earlier chapters we now need to have a look at the array of terms we use when using fractions.

Language used in relation to fractions	
Whole numbers	Lowest terms
Half, quarter, third (the naming of fractions)	Denominator
Equal parts	Numerator
Out of	Lowest common denominator
Left over or remainder	Highest common factor
Vulgar	Top heavy
Comparisons such as more than, less than, equal to, the same as	Equivalent
	Proper/improper
Cancel, reduce or simplify	Mixed numbers

Source: McLeoad and Newmarch (2006)

Calculating body mass index

At this stage it is worth revisiting Edward's story and working out his BMI using a calculation that does use the skills identified when working with fractions in the form of the BMI formula. Whilst there are many calculators for BMI available online it is worth knowing how to calculate it manually.

$$\text{BMI (kg/m}^2) = \frac{\text{Weight (in kg)}}{\text{Height (in metres)}^2}$$

Squaring a number (indicated by the 2 after the bracket i.e. square^2) means multiplying the number by itself.

BMI ranges for the adult population.

BMI (kg/m²)	Weight defined
Below 18.5	Underweight
18.5–24.9	Normal
25–29.9	Overweight
30–39.9	Obese (Class I & II)
Above 40	Very obese (Class III)

Source: Adapted from WHO (2004) data for the adult population

This is the information used for the adult population. With children the BMI is then plotted on a percentile growth chart to then categorise which category they fit into. Have a look at these charts on the ONE resource.

Section 3 Child growth standards at the World Health Organisation can be accessed at: http://www.who.int/childgrowth/en/

Go to http://www.who.int/growthref/bmifa_boys_z_5_19_labels.pdf to have a look at the chart that will be used to assess the degree of obesity for Nathan – WHO reference data 2007.

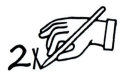

Using the formula calculate Nathan's BMI (to one decimal place) and the category he fits into the adult categories. How does this equate and differ when recorded on the children's growth standards/BMI chart?

There are more practice examples on the website – Activity 4B

PERCENTAGES

Per cent means per hundred so percentages are everything to do with parts of a hundred in the same way that a fraction is a part of 1.

It has its own symbol, that is, % and it is well recognisable by all especially in a shopping context where 20% off the price or, even better, 75% off has a clear meaning for the shopper. Most marking systems will award marks in percentages (as well as alphanumeric scales A, B, C etc.). Percentages are an easy way to represent health-related data, that is, 35% of children within 50 miles of Arch Mede Hospital are overweight. 100% means the whole amount where 50% would be one-half of it (½) and 25% would be one-quarter (¼) and 10% would be one-tenth (1/10).

Also look back to the Eatwell plate and consider whether the percentage values have a clearer meaning than the fractions?

How to turn a percentage into a fraction?

You convert a percentage into a fraction by placing the percentage number over 100 in the following fashion.

$$\frac{35}{100}$$

This can clearly be cancelled down or simplified by dividing by 5 to get 7/20.

How to find a percentage of a number?

For example, to find 35% of 175, convert the percentage into a fraction, that is, 35/100 and multiply by the total number, that is, 175 (which you can also present as a fraction by placing it over a denominator of one to make the multiplication of two fractions look more balanced and equal).

$$\frac{35}{100} \times \frac{175}{1} = 61.25$$

Have a look at the sum first – can you simplify the fractions in any way?

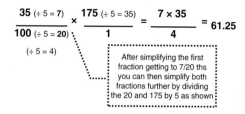

$$\frac{35 \ (\div 5 = 7)}{100 \ (\div 5 = 20)} \times \frac{175 \ (\div 5 = 35)}{1} = \frac{7 \times 35}{4} = 61.25$$

$(\div 5 = 4)$

After simplifying the first fraction getting to 7/20 ths you can then simplify both fractions further by dividing the 20 and 175 by 5 as shown

As shown in the figure above, from 35/100 you get 7/20. Then you can also cross-simplify and divide the 20 and 175 by 5 to get 7/4 × 35 = 245/4 = 61.25.

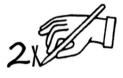

Have a go at the further examples:

- 53% of 625
- 75% of 95
- 31% of 350
- 12% of 500

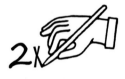

When calculating a baby's expected weight you need to know the birth weight and baby's age in weeks. You also have to remember that a baby may lose and then regain up to one-tenth (10%) of their body weight in the first 2 weeks of life.

Work out how much weight (in grams) both Edward and Nathan lost during the first 2 weeks of their lives?

How to turn a percentage into a decimal amount?

To turn a percentage into a decimal amount you need to first turn the percentage into a fraction and then divide the top number by the bottom number (which will be a 100 so it is a simple division and a move of two decimal places to the left) as demonstrated here.

i.e. 35% = 35/100 = 0.35

Examples of percentages in nursing practice: Solutions, lotions and potions.

1. Solutions

If you have a good look at the solutions used in practice you will see that percentage concentrations are usually expressed in three different ways, that is, weight in volume (w/v), weight in weight (w/w) or volume in volume (v/v).

What usually causes confusion is that we are relating weight and volume together so we are not working with the same units, that is, grams and millilitres in the weight in volume formulation, which applies to intravenous fluids such as 0.9% w/v sodium chloride.

This means that 0.9 g of sodium chloride is dissolved in 100 mL of water. If we want to find out how much sodium chloride there is in a 500 mL bag you need to do the following calculation.

0.9/100 and multiply by 500 which gives you 4.5 g OR just multiply 0.9 g by 5 because you need a 5:1 ratio of sodium chloride.

Note: Generally we work with the idea that 1 litre of water weights 1 kilogram so 1 mL will equal 1 g (please note this is a generalisation and only is accurate when talking about water, though for the purposes of these calculations it can be used).

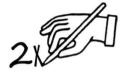

Have a go at the following:

- How much glucose is there in 250 mL of 5% w/v glucose solution?
- How much potassium chloride is there in 10 mL of 15% w/v potassium chloride?

Another worked example: Pi (from Chapter 7) is admitted with ketoacidosis and we may need to give him some glucose solution and we want to know how much glucose he is getting. So if 200 mL of a 20% glucose solution is given to him:

- What do we know?

20% solution contains 20 g in 100 mL of water.

Turn the percentage into a fraction and multiply by the volume given.

$20/100 \times 20 = 40$ g.

We can also work on this the other way around and a different perspective, that is, if 50 g of glucose is prescribed as an IV injection, what volume of a 20% solution will we need for the dose?

We know that 20 g is in a 100 mL (to make a 20% solution) so we can use various methods to calculate how much we need for the dose, which takes us neatly to a discussion around ratios.

Method 1 To use fractions and percentages we know that 20 g = 100 mL so we need to find what 50 g = ? So we need to divide 50 by 20 and multiply by 100 = 250 mL.

Method 2 Alternatively, you could find out what 1 mL is equal to (i.e. 20 divided by 100 = 0.2 g) and then divide 50 g by this amount, that is, $50 \div 20/100 = 50 \times 100/20 = 250$ mL (remember how to divide using fractions or use the decimal form).

For a volume/volume solution we work in exactly the same way, so if a drug is supplied as a 20% v/v solution we know we have 20 mL of drug for every 100 mL of solution.

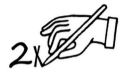

Have a go at some more with Magic Medicine A which is supplied as a 15% solution: How much solution do you need to get?

- 7.5 g of Magic Medicine A
- 22.5 g of Magic Medicine A
- 45 g of Magic Medicine A?

2. Local anaesthetics

Here are some more examples using a commonly used local anaesthetic:

Lidocaine

Lidocaine is usually supplied in 0.5%, 1% and 2% solutions, so it is important to understand how much of the local anaesthetic a child is being given.

If 1 mL of a 1% solution of lidocaine has been given to a child – how much has he received?

1 g of drug in 100 mL = 1000 mg in 100 mL = 10 mg per mL, so the child has been given 10 mg of lidocaine.

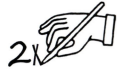

Have a go at the practice examples? Fill in the blanks in the following table:

Lidocaine	mg per mL
0.1%	
0.2%	
0.5%	
1%	10
2%	
5%	

At this point we could also consider topical anaesthetics such as Ametop and EMLA creams. Look them up in the BNF and identify what percentage of local anaesthetic and dose the child is getting when applied as per manufacturers recommendations.

3. Fluid management

As mentioned in the previous chapter we sometimes need to calculate a percentage of the total maintenance fluids that will be administered to avoid the risk of circulatory overload, for example for children with head trauma.

Whilst Nathan did not have any intravenous fluids administered whilst he was in theatre let us use him as an example just in case he might do post-operatively.

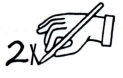

Nathan weighs 42.5 kg so first calculate his maintenance fluids, then the hourly rate and then work out:

- 60% of total daily maintenance fluids and hourly rate
- 75% of total daily maintenance fluids and hourly rate

Investigations

On Day 2 of his admission the decision is made to perform a sweat test on Edward, following close observation and fluid balance monitoring on Day 1. A sweat test is the gold standard for the diagnosis of cystic fibrosis and is carried out by clinical chemistry departments. It needs to be carried out accurately and is fairly straightforward to perform and is painless.

It is performed on an infant's right arm or thigh, where gauze pads are applied to the skin; one of which is soaked in pilocarpine which makes the skin sweat and the other in saline. Electrodes are placed over the gauze and produced a mild electric current, after 5–10 minutes which causes tingling only. The second part of the test involves cleaning the area and collecting the sweat on a piece of paper or gauze and 30 minutes later, collected sweat is sent to the laboratory.

ACB (2003) make the following comments based on best evidence:

- A sweat chloride concentration of greater than 60 mmol/L supports the diagnosis of CF.
- Intermediate chloride concentration of 40–60 mmol/L is suggestive but not diagnostic of CF.
- A sweat chloride of less than 40 mmol/L is normal and there is a low probability of CF.
- Sodium should not be interpreted without a chloride result.

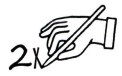

The sweat test involves a simple measure of chloride concentration in mmol/L. Can you think of any investigations that measure numbers or amounts in percentages?

Go to the website and practise some more percentage calculations by doing Activity 4C.

RATIO OR PROPORTION?

Actually defining the difference between what is ratio and what is proportion is not very easy though what follows is an attempt to do this in a way that is meaningful to nursing practice.

Ratio

A ratio can be defined very simply and easily as part to part.

A ratio is the relationship between two or more quantities. When diluting juice, for example, for every part concentrate we need 4 parts water. This could be written as 1 to 4, 4 for every 1 or 4 to every 1. It is here that literacy becomes the key to understanding the nursing problem. We need to clarify the meaning of the words used where 1 **IN** 10 means 1 part **IN** a total of 10 parts. Whilst what does 1:10 and 1 **TO** 10 then mean? 1 part is added to 10 parts making a total of 11 parts.

Juice diluted to 1:4.

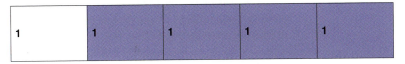

Examples of ratios in nursing practice

1. Adrenaline (epinephrine)

Adrenaline (epinephrine) is a commonly used drug used in resuscitation situations usually involving allergic or circulatory failure. It is supplied in strengths of 1 in 1000 and 1 in 10,000.

As you can clearly see there is the potential for errors to be made in relation to the 'zero' and the second characteristic that should be obvious is the fact that this is a ratio where there is 1 part adrenaline in 999 parts of solution or 1 part in 9999 of solution.

There is 1 g of adrenaline in 1000 mL of solution = 1000 mg in 1000 mL = 1 mg per 1 mL.

In the 1 in 100,000 formulation

1 g in 10,000 mL

1000 mg in 10,000 mL

0.1 mg in 1 mL which = 100 micrograms per mL.

Clearly this then is a weaker solution and therefore is the most suitable for use in children's practice.

2. Child growth and development

The upper-to-lower body segment ratio changes with growth. Normally, the ratio at birth is 1:7, the ratio at age 3 is 1:3, and the ratio by age 7 becomes 1. The lower body segment is measured from the symphysis pubis to the floor.

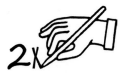

You are doing experiments and making magic potions with the play staff and Nathan in the playroom and the potion is made up of three solutions A, B and C. To make the potion change colour and turn a nice shade of ghoulish green you need 10 mL of A, 20 mL of B and 5 mL of C.

- What is the ratio of A:B, B:C and C:A?
- The total amount of A + B + C is 35 mL and Nathan has decided to prepare 87.5 mL – how many millilitres of A, B and C will you need to prepare this amount?

PROPORTION

Proportion can be defined as a part to whole.

A portion or part in its relation to the whole; a comparative part, a share - one part concentrate in every five parts. From the GCSE curriculum (AQA, 2006) the definition for proportion is basically that fractions, decimals and percentages are three different ways of expressing a proportion of something.

Clearly we could end up with major errors when diluting medications in particular if we do not understand these mathematical concepts.

PROBABILITY

Whilst we are not discussing probability in this chapter it does sort of fit here in terms of the probability that Nathan has inherited the CF gene from his parents who we now find out are both carriers of the gene and percentages come into the outcome, where parents ask for the chance of having another child with cystic fibrosis.

Probability is the branch of statistics that allows you to calculate how likely something is to happen and give this happening a numerical value, that is, when tossing a coin there are two possible outcomes – whether it will land on a head or tail so there is a 1 in 2 chance it will land on a head (or 50% chance or a fraction ½ or 0.5 as a decimal), (Usborne Illustrated Dictionary, 2006).

	Mum Carrier of CF gene		Dad Carrier of CF gene	
Child 1 Affected 1 in 4 25% risk	**Child 2** Carrier of CF gene 1 in 2 50% chance of being a carrier		**Child 3** Unaffected 1 in 2 50% chance of being a carrier	**Child 4** 1 in 4 25% Unaffected

In relation to Nathan's siblings who have a different father the risk of them being carriers is.

Mum Carrier of CF gene		Dad No CF	
Child 1 Unaffected Carrier of CF gene	Child 2 Unaffected Carrier of CF gene	Child 3 Unaffected Not a carrier	Child 4 Unaffected Not a carrier

Numeracy related to case scenarios

So what about Edward and Nathan who illustrate the two opposite ends of the spectrum with respect to being underweight and overweight? To comprehend the meaning of the numerical information that we need to deal with it is vital to have an understanding of the physiological processes that are taking place in relation to both the children. Whilst nutritional information is the domain of the dietician in relation to the detail of specific dietary advice it does fall to us as nurses to understand and explain to parents, that is, why Edward is not feeding well and putting on weight and why Nathan is overweight and unhealthy in both scenarios as guided by the ESC's from the NMC (2010).

Though it is obvious to state, a regular supply of dietary energy is essential for life, and is required as fuel for the many different metabolic processes that are going on in our bodies including growth and development. Daily energy requirements vary widely from one individual to the next, due to factors such as sex, body size, bodyweight, environment and physical activity levels. Energy is obtained, from the food and drink we consume, by oxidation of carbohydrate, fat and protein, known as macronutrients. The amount of energy that each of these macronutrients provides varies.

Macronutrient	Energy provided
Fat	9 kcal (37 kJ) per gram
Protein	4 kcal (17 kJ) per gram
Carbohydrate	3.75 kcal (16 kJ) per gram

How is energy intake measured?

Going back to the information on units in Chapter 2 you will realise that energy intake is measured in joules (J) (or kilojoules (kJ)) but most of us may be more used to working in calories or kilocalories.

1 kilojoule (kJ) = 1000 joules

1 megajoule (MJ) = 1,000,000 joules

1 kilocalorie (kcal) = 1000 calories or 1 calorie

To convert from one unit to another:

1 kcal = 4.184 kJ, so a 1000 kcal diet provides 4.184 MJ or 4184 kJ

1 MJ = 239 kcal

Energy expenditure is the sum (addition) of the basal metabolic rate (BMR) (the amount of energy expended while at rest at a neutral temperature and whilst fasting), the thermic effect of food (or known as dietary-induced thermogenesis) and the energy expended in movement and exercise. A substantial proportion of total energy expenditure is accounted for by BMR, which is determined principally by body mass and body composition both of which vary with age and sex (see below for date related to boys and girls). The actual amount of energy needed is a very individual thing and depends on their BMR and how active they are.

Basal metabolic rate

The BMR is the rate at which a person uses energy to maintain the basic functions of the body, such as respiration, cardiac function and keeping warm, when at complete rest. An average adult will use around 1.1 kcal each minute just maintaining these functions and BMR varies from one person to the next as already stated.

Children are different and infants and young children tend to have a proportionately high BMR for their size due to their rapid growth and development as already mentioned in earlier chapters. Children need more energy intake due to this higher metabolic rate and they also have reduced fat stores meaning they have less resistance when coping with illness, trauma, infection or metabolic stress (RCN, 2006).

Have a look at the additional information about physical activity levels related to BMR in Section 3 of the ONE resource, including formulae that can be used to calculate it.

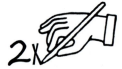

When thinking about the use of units can you see how important it is to utilise MJ rather than KJ to avoid making errors in relation to the use of zeroes?

Energy requirements for growth and development

Calorific intake to assure adequate intake in a normal infant is 100–110 kcal/kg/day for the first half year (6 months) and 100 kcal/kg/day for the second half of the first year. Beyond 10 kg, 50 kcal/kg/day is required until a weight of 20 kg is achieved. Beyond 20 kg, 20 kcal/kg/day is necessary.

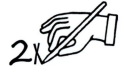

Convert the above energy requirements from kilocalories into kilojoules and megajoules.

Age/weight	kcal/kg/day	kJ/kg/day	MJ/kg/day
0–6 months	100–110	418.40–460.24	0.4184–0.46
6–12 months	100		
10–20 kg	50		
>20 kg	20		

Then calculate Edward's energy requirements per day based on his estimated weight of 7 kg.

Why is this information important?

The RCN (2006) position statement on Malnutrition, to reinforce the NMC (2010) competencies state that nurses who work with children and young people have an important role in identifying whether children are at risk of malnutrition and monitoring it.

The British Association of Parenteral and Enteral Nutrition (BAPEN) defines undernutrition as a deficiency of energy and/or nutrients and vice versa for overnutrition, that is a result of excess of nutrients. Whilst we do not use the same tools used in adult nursing we already have the necessary tools in our toolkit to monitor and screen for malnourishment, that is, weighing the child in hospital (once weekly), measuring length/height where there is concern and plotting measurement on a centile chart. Whilst BMI is an important measure, as with monitoring weight it should be viewed in context with other parameters over time. In adult healthcare screening tools for malnutrition have long been introduced which is also happening in children's areas. Have a look at the links to find out more.

BAPEN and link to MUST tools for screening adult patients:
http://www.bapen.org.uk/screening-for-malnutrition/must/introducing-must

A link to a paediatric version of this tool:
http://www.nutritioncare.scot.nhs.uk/pyms.aspx

With respect to managing the environment for eating and drinking, nurses should be skilled at weighing and measuring height, be able to support breastfeeding mothers and identify problems when they occur, know how to select, prepare and handle age-appropriate foods and formulas, know how to select correct portion sizes for children, give advice around feeding patterns and mealtimes and know how to give weaning advice within a cultural and social context. They should also recognise the visual signs of malnutrition (RCN, 2006). These are all skills utilised when caring for both Edward and Nathan.

Numbers, as hopefully identified, have a clear role in being able to do this effectively and give the support and advice that parent and children need. Chapter 7 will discuss some of these issues further in relation to the management of diabetes mellitus.

Whilst we are not dieticians and will not be offering very detailed nutritional information to our patients, we are in the position of having to offer health promotion advice in relation to both Edward and Nathan.

Have a think about the following using the information offered on dairy products on the ONE resource:

- What advice would you offer Edward's mum when she asks about which infant formula she should be giving to him, why cow's milk is not recommended until he is over 1 and how to wean him?
- WHO recommends eating a minimum of 400 g per day of fruit and vegetables – how would you quantify this when asked by Nathan to explain what this looks like?

Outcomes in relation to Edward and Nathan

Edward is diagnosed with cystic fibrosis and Nathan does have dental surgery done and leaves hospital with referrals to be followed up by dietician, paediatrician and school nursing team. Edward's mum and dad have the opportunity to talk to the dietician as well as all the members of the multidisciplinary team, particularly the Consultant paediatrician, whereas the nurses caring for Nathan only have the opportunity to give some advice, offer some leaflets and ensure that referrals have been made as already discussed, though both dad and Nathan are happy with the information that has been made available for them to discuss with mum at home.

CONCLUDING COMMENTS

This chapter has explored the world of parts of the whole number, focusing in on the use of fractions (including decimals), ratio and proportion as important numeracy skills to possess as we move to using nursing formulae, where we put all the parts together in more complex numerical operations, in the next chapter. The numerical operations have been linked to practice using small parts or episodes of Euler and Newton family stories, which hopefully have set a context for acquiring competence in these skills.

Chapter 5

PUTTING THE PIECES TOGETHER – A FORMULA FOR CHILDREN'S NURSES

Numeracy in Children's Nursing, First Edition. Arija Parker
© 2015 John Wiley & Sons, Ltd. Published 2015 by John Wiley & Sons Ltd.

LEARNING FOCUS

Putting the numerical pieces together to use in a formula context
This chapter will focus in on the skills already covered; basic operations, use of fractions, percentages, ratios and proportion combined with the use of a formula to calculate medication amounts for children and young people. What should become evident is that you do not have to use a formula and in matching with the numeracy practice in other chapters, what will be offered are many suggestions for how to accurately calculate the correct amount of medication to be administered to a child or a young person.

LEARNING OUTCOMES

By the end of this chapter you should be able to:

- Refresh your knowledge on pharmacological principles as they apply to children and young people including how to administer medications to children safely and competently
- Identify which numerical method you want to use when calculating medicine dosages, whether it be a formula or alternative method, in line with the approach taken in earlier chapters
- Continue to practice calculation in relation to the most common medications used in children and young people's nursing practice

CASE SCENARIO 6

Alice Agnesi (aged 2½ years) has been admitted to the Children's unit with a chest infection. She is accompanied by her mother, who will be residing with her. She has a 4-year-old brother who is being cared for by her grandmother. She weighs 12.6 kg on admission.

Hospital number	AMH2014-06
Ward number	Beta Ward 2 (The children's unit)

Temperature	Pulse	Blood pressure	Respirations	CRT	Sa O$_2$	Pain score	PEWS score
38.4°C	159 bpm	$\frac{111}{66}$	45 per minute	<2 seconds	92%	0	3

Alice's blood results on admission

Urea and electrolytes		Normal values	Full blood count & differential		Normal values
Sodium	142	136–143 mmol/L	Haemoglobin	13	13.8 g/dL
Potassium	4.9	4.1–5.6 mmol/L	Platelets	300	200–500 × 10^9/L
Chloride	101	98–106 mmol/L	White cell count	13.5	4–12 × 10^9/L
Creatinine	75	<80 µmol/L	Neutrophils	8	1.5–7 × 10^9/L
Urea	5.5	2.5–6.7 mmol/L	Lymphocytes	9.1	5–8.5 × 10^9/L
OTHER BLOOD TESTS TAKEN ON ADMISSION			Basophils	0.04	0.04 × 10^9/L
CRP	53	No normal reference range	Monocytes	0.9	0.7–1.5 × 10^9/L
			Eosinophils	0.2	0.2 × 10^9/L

Source: Normal ranges taken from Skinner (2005) and the ranges used from the original case scenario examples.

Function of white blood cells – a brief description

We commonly measure a white blood cell count as part of a full blood count for children and young people for a variety of reasons and the medical staff might then proceed, as in Alice's case, to request a differential white cell count, which will offer a more detailed assessment of the type of white blood cell that is present. Each white blood cell or leukocyte has its own function and is present in a different percentage amount in the blood as already discussed in Chapter 4. What follows is a brief description of these functions so that you can start thinking about what might be the causative agent in Alice's presentation with the clear signs and symptoms of a chest infection.

Neutrophils are an important line of defence against invading organisms and are the most abundant of the white cells. When explaining what they do to children you would probably describe them as the 'soldiers' in terms of the defensive role they have in the human body. They destroy invading organisms by phagocytoses, so a raised neutrophil count is an indication of a normal body response to invasive agents.

Lymphocytes are the second most abundant of the white blood cells and first line of defence against disease and invading organisms. They come in two types – T-lymphocytes and β-lymphocytes – and they are responsible for initiating and regulating the immune response by the production of antibodies and cytokines.

Basophils launch into action in relation to allergic reactions and also offer some defence to worm parasites. The immunoglobulin IgE has a natural attraction to a basophil so when it comes into contact with the allergen the basophil responds by releasing histamine and other chemicals to mediate the allergic response.

Monocytes respond to inflammation in the tissues and will be increased in response to infections such as sub-acute bacterial endocarditis, tuberculosis, hepatitis, malaria and infectious mononucleosis.

Eosinophils have the job of dealing with allergic and parasitic conditions and will be raised if the child has been admitted with an exacerbation of asthma, hay fever, food or medicine sensitivity or parasitic infections such as roundworm as one example of many.

To identify the presence of infection or disease we may also monitor erythrocyte sedimentation rate (ESR), though in Alice's case a C-reactive protein (CRP) was performed which is a good way of detecting the presence of infection in a more accurate way, because it changes more rapidly than ESR and levels are increased up to several hundred times following an acute infective or non-infective inflammatory response.

What is the numerical data in the form of Alice's blood results and her observations giving you clues about following what would be your initial assessment of ABCDE when she is admitted to the ward and into your care?

Have a look at one of Alice's PEWS charts in Section 1.

From her prescription chart the medicines administered are: four hourly salbutamol nebulisers, co-amoxiclav 380 mg IV at 07.00, 15.00 and 23.00, paracetamol 190 mg and Oxygen 40% via mask initially and then 28% via nasal cannula. This chapter will focus on the medications administered to Alice whilst in hospital.

CASE SCENARIO 7

8-year-old Luke Lovelace has been admitted to Beta Ward, via A&E, with a painful left elbow sustained after playing football. Following an X-ray, it was diagnosed as a supracondylar fracture of the left humerus. On admission to A&E at 20.10 hours, he was given 0.2 mL of intranasal diamorphine and was then cannulated and given a bolus of normal saline 240 mL intravenously (he had not had anything to eat or drink since mid-afternoon). He was then commenced on intravenous fluids at 65 mL per hour, because he was being starved, so Nil By Mouth, and awaiting theatre. He was taken to Beta Ward 2 at midnight and was eventually taken to theatre at 08.30 in the morning, where manipulation and insertion of a K-wire and application of plaster of Paris backslab and collar and cuff took place. Back on the ward he recovered well from this first time experience of fracturing a bone and being in hospital and was discharged a day later. He was weighed in A&E – 27 kg.

Hospital number	AMH2014-07
Ward number	Beta Ward 2 (The children's unit)

Temperature	Pulse	Blood pressure	Respirations	CRT	Pain score	PEWS score
36.6°C	108 bpm	$\frac{109}{60}$	30 per minute	<2 seconds	4	1

From Luke's prescription chart the medicines administered were: cefuroxime 750 mg (for surgical prophylaxis), 12.5 mg of diclofenac sodium PR and 725 mg of paracetamol (given IV over 15 minutes) in theatre. Paracetamol was supplied as 10 mg/mL and diluted to a concentration of 1 mg/1 mL with sodium chloride 0.9%. Postoperatively he was prescribed paracetamol and ibuprofen.

This chapter will focus in on Luke's pain management and the range of analgesics that were (or could have been) administered to him.

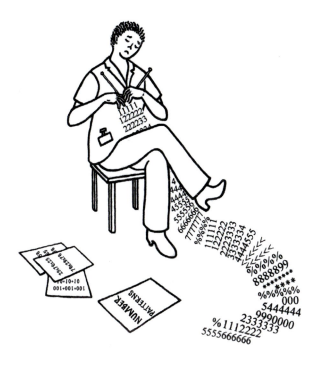

INTRODUCTION

This chapter will focus on medicine calculations and the numeracy skills needed to ensure safe administration of medicines to children and young people. All the numeracy skills explored to date will be combined into the use of formulae that are frequently used in children's nursing practice. As already stated there are many methods that can be used to calculate so you do not have to use a formula – these alternatives will be outlined throughout this chapter. Principles of safe medication administration will be covered briefly to reinforce the safety message that will be a core theme within this chapter. Whilst the two case scenarios outlined above will be the focus of this chapter, the prescriptions of other children from earlier chapters will be utilised as extra exemplars. The more common medications will be discussed in this chapter. The next chapter will progress to more complex medication calculations from a neonatal perspective.

The numeracy skills to be covered in this chapter include interpreting written data from prescription charts, use of formulae that are underpinned by the numeracy skills already covered in earlier chapters and calculating medicine dosages prescribed in different formulations and via different routes.

Setting the context

The NMC standards for pre-registration nursing education (2010) state in domain 3 for children's nursing: Nursing practice and decision-making

'All nurses must practise safely by being aware of the correct use, limitations and hazards of common interventions, including nursing activities, treatments, the calculation and administration of medicines, and the use of medical devices and equipment. The nurse must be able to evaluate their use, report any concerns promptly through appropriate channels and modify care where necessary to maintain safety. They must contribute to the collection of local and national data and formulation of policy on risks, hazards and adverse outcomes.' (NMC, 2010, p. 45)

And, in relation to children in particular 6.1:

'Children's nurses must have numeracy skills for medicines management, assessment, measuring, monitoring and recording which recognise the particular vulnerability of infants and young children in relation accurate medicines calculation.' (NMC, 2010)

With respect to the Essential Skills Clusters 33–41 (NMC, 2010) the summary of skills needed and included are as follows:

- Competence in relation to medication-related calculation, that is, tablets/capsules, liquid medicines, injections and IV infusions (unit dose, sub and multiple unit dose), complex calculations and SI conversions
- Working within legal and ethical frameworks that underpin safe and effective medicine management

- Working as part of team to ensure holistic care (including distraction and complementary therapies which in relation to children's nursing and in the context of this chapter would include play and distraction)
- Safe and effective practice in medicines management by knowing the actions, risk and benefits of medicines (ESC 36)
- Safely ordering, receiving, storing and disposing of medicines (including controlled medicines in any setting (ESC 37)
- Administering of medicines safely and in a timely manner (ESC 38)
- Maintaining accurate record of medications administered (EC 39)
- Working in partnership with patients and clients (ESC 40)
- Using and evaluating up-to-date knowledge (ESC 41)

For registered nurses and students this is all set within the context of the NMC guidance for medication administration. The scope of this book does not allow for in-depth examination of all the details of these requirements, which is why the focus is very much on the competences needed for student nurses in training, though it is worth reflecting on your knowledge of these standards and having a look and read of them. The link to the NMC (2010) Standards for medicines management is: http://www.nmcuk.org/Documents/Standards/nmcStandardsForMedicinesManagementBooklet.pdf

PHARMACOLOGY AND CHILDREN AND YOUNG PEOPLE: HOW MEDICINES WORK

Whilst the principles of pharmacology are not the core focus of the book, which is all about the numbers part of the process, it is worth reiterating that we need to take a holistic approach to the administration of medicines. This then ensures that nurses have a deeper knowledge of anatomy and physiology, how medicines work and so what the numbers actually mean within the context of this complex and vitally important nursing skill. Again this is about recognizing the close relationship between literacy and numeracy where you need to understand both to be able to practice safely and with care.

Why do we need to understand this process?

There are many reasons which include the need to understand the underlying rationale for the treatment plans prescribed for children and young people in our care, ensuring safety and reducing risk. This guarantees competence as well as ensures that we have the knowledge that can then be passed on to more junior colleagues and, most importantly, to children and their families when teaching and educating them about medicines, treatments and regimes.

The key pharmacological processes that we need to be knowledgeable about are pharmacokinetics and pharmacodynamics. The use of the word 'drug' and 'medicine' is used interchangeable though the keyword 'medicine' is used mostly as the preferred term, because the word 'drug' tends to have negative connotations whereas a medicine is seen to be more therapeutic.

Pharmacokinetics is 'what the body does to the drug' or the study of how a drug (or medicine) is absorbed, distributed, metabolised and excreted. Nurses need to understated these processes to ensure safe and effective therapeutic administration of medicines to patients. The way children respond to medicines is going to be very different from adults, which is why nurse or healthcare professionals caring for children need to be very aware of the special considerations we need to afford children when administering medications, including the physiological differences, as well as developmental differences.

Pharmacodynamics refers to 'what the medicine does to the body' and looks at the relationship between medicine concentration at the site of medicine action and the effect that results including the time course and intensity of therapeutic and adverse (side) effects.

Absorption is the process by which fluids and other substances, that is, nutrients and medicines are taken up by the body tissues, where the main site of absorption is the small intestine. The rate of absorption will be determined by route of administration, where it is given and the solubility of the medicine. To illustrate these points if in liquid form as in the case of giving paracetamol to children, the medicine will be absorbed more rapidly, uptake will be better if the child is generally warm and contact time – where for an oral medication you will need to think about gastric emptying and gut motility, that is, if a child has gastroenteritis like Tommy in Chapter 3, where absorption of oral medications will be reduced. Alice is having salbutamol nebulisers, where such a large surface area like the lungs will ensure that the nebulised medication will be absorbed very efficiently if Alice tolerates the mask and time it takes to administer the medicine.

Clearly the problems we have in administering certain medicines to children will have an impact on how they are absorbed, that is, the need to use liquid formulations as opposed to tablets. We also have to be aware of the potential problems of high sugar content in some syrups (which improve the taste, so children will take them, though cause dental caries), as well as use of tartrazine, which may cause hyperactivity in some children. In neonatal setting medicines not available in suitable concentrations necessitate the use of complex dilutions thus increasing the risk of medicine errors, which will be discussed in much greater detail in Chapter 6.

Other issues to think about in relation to children according to Kelly (2001) include:

- Medicines that rely on enzyme activity will demonstrate variable bioavailability in children, where adult levels are achieved at various ages

- Reduced levels of gut flora will increase the bioavailability of medicines like digoxin, so will need to be used with care with children
- In relation to topical administration – children have thinner stratum corneum – absorption is increased 2.7-fold in the newborn and young infant. Medicines like corticosteroids will be absorbed excessively so use with care

Distribution is the way in which the medicine is transported to the source tissues and is dependent on circulatory function: core organs have the best distribution and the skin the worst distribution. This will be affected by cardiac output, regional blood flow, how the medicine binds to plasma protein among other factors. The key difference with children is that as discussed in earlier chapters infants' body weight has a higher percentage of water than older children or adults, so water-soluble medicines are diluted to a greater extent therefore higher doses may be required to produce the required plasma concentration and serum albumin and total protein concentrations are decreased during early infancy up to 1 year.

Metabolism is the first stage of medicine clearance whereby a medicine is chemically altered to aid elimination from the body, where the primary site of medicine metabolism is the liver though other organs are involved, that is, lungs, kidneys, blood and intestines. With children, the key difference from adults is that as a result of metabolic immaturity, medicines will be cleared by the liver more slowly so the medicine therapy needs to be closely monitored.

Excretion involves excreting the metabolites of the medicine from the body via kidneys for the most part. The rate of excretion will depend on the type of medicine, where again the immaturity of the neonate and infant may necessitate the need for reduced doses of some medicines, which we need to be aware of.

This creates an acronym ADME, which is a useful way of remembering the processes as well as remembering that responses to medicines are not always predictable and vary much in individuals from child to child, adult to adult.

Reintroducing fractions and pharmacodynamics

Half-life of a medicine

- Time taken for the activity of a medicine to reduce to half its original level
- A steady state concentration is achieved when the amount of medicine eliminated over a specific time interval is equal to the amount of medicine entering the plasma at the same time interval
- Steady state – the medicine in the plasma remains constant
- Medicine plasma levels reach a therapeutic level after 4–5 half-lives from the time of initial dose
- Dosages should be given with every passing half-life to achieve a steady state concentration
- In the previous example the repeat doses should be given four hourly, that is, a 500 mg medicine with a half-life of 4 hours enters the blood stream at 10 AM. At 2 PM it will have a plasma concentration of 250 mg. At 6 PM it will have a plasma concentration of 125 mg

This covers the basic underpinnings of healthcare knowledge of how medicines work and why we need to know this. So let us now proceed to the administration process and start to focus in on the numbers involved.

The prescription chart

This section will clearly and concisely cover the essential aspects in relation to interpreting the prescription chart. Clearly this has to be done in advance of starting the checking and calculation process. As already mentioned early on in this book this is the aspect of children's nursing practice where numerical errors frequently occur. How can we avoid these errors? There are many healthcare professionals involved in this multidisciplinary activity – the prescriber (who can be a doctor, dentist, midwife or a nurse amongst many others), the pharmacist, the nurse (or person who gives the medicine) as well as the patient themselves who may be self-administering the medicine as well as taking it.

From the literature reviewed and from practice guidelines these 'rights' exist in a variety of forms and numbers ranging from 4–10. For the purposes of this book the Arch Mede Hospital 6 rights will be discussed.

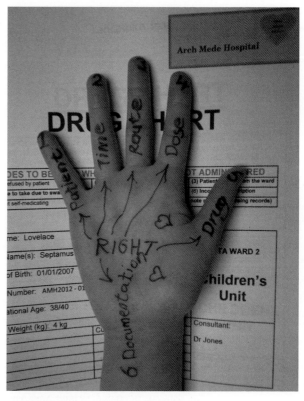

The rights related to medicine administration.

The rights

Right medicine – check that the medicine is prescribed by using generic or non-proprietary name (not the trade, patented or brand name), that is, salbutamol not Ventolin, paracetamol not Calpol). It is also important to check dosage strength, that is, paracetamol 120 mg in 5 mL or 250 mg in 5 mL as one example.

Right dose – check the dose – the prescriber and the giver of the medication both have a legal responsibility of knowing what the correct dose is. In children's nursing, medicines are prescribed on the basis of weight so ensure that the child's weight is recorded on the prescription chart also.

Right route – check whether the medicine is to be given orally, parenterally or cutaneously (see abbreviations commonly used below, that is, p.o., IV etc.)

Right time – check when and how often they should be given, where thinking about the time aspect should also prompt you to think to check expiry date!

Right patient –check verbally by asking the child and/or parent/carer (name and date of birth) and visually (patient name band against prescription chart as well as looking at the child himself or herself). At the same time ensure that you educate the child and parent/carer by explaining what you are giving as well as why medication is being given.

Right documentation – check the prescription chart is legible, check for allergies, check for any specific actions you may need to do before giving medication, that is, checking observations and ensure that you sign that you have given the medicine.

Again it is worth reflecting on and developing a personal approach to remembering the 'rights' or putting some order or structure to the checking process, where adding extra rights such as the right to refuse, right attitude and right expiry date might make the process more meaningful for you. The table below will also give you some more information in relation to the 'rights' discussed above.

A full colour version of the picture above is included on the online resource for you to adapt and download to 'give you a hand' as a prompt.

The language of prescription charts

Before you can understand what medicine you need to administer you need to understand the language of a prescription chart. Have a look at some of the common abbreviations.

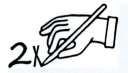

What language are they written in and why do we use this language?

Common abbreviations used in prescribing practice.

Abbreviation	Latin meaning	English meaning	Comments
a.c.	ante cibum	before meals	
ad lib	add libitum	use as much as you desire; freely	
alt. h.	alternis horis	every other hour	
Amp		ampoule	
Aq	aqua	water	
bis	bis	twice	
b.d./b.i.d.	bis in die		Twelve hourly
Cib	cibus	with food	
dieb.alt.	diebus alternis	every other day	
gtt(s)	guttae(s)	drop(s)	
h, hr	hora	Hour	
mane	Mane	in the morning	
m.d.u.	more dicto utendus	to be used as directed	
neb	nebula	a spray	
noct.	nocte	at night	
Od	omne in die	everyday/once daily	
per	Per	by or through	
p.c.	post cibum	after meals	
p.o.	per os	by mouth or orally	
p.r.	per rectum	rectally	
prn	pro re nata	as needed	
q.d.s. OR q.i.d.	quater die sumendus OR quattuor in die	four times a day	Six hourly
SL		sublingually or under the tongue	
stat	statim	immediately	
supp	suppositorium	suppository	
susp		suspension	
Syr	syrupus	syrup	
Tab	tabella	tablet	
t.d.s.	ter die sumendum	three times a day	Eight hourly
t.i.d.	ter in die	three times a day	

According to Muldoon (1916) the ancient language of Latin should find 'present day use in chemical and pharmaceutical nomenclature' and particularly in the writing of prescriptions for the following reasons:

- It is a dead language so there will be no increase in vocabulary, where words will not change
- It is a universal language – in theory, at the time, understood by all educated persons in all parts of the world (remembering that he was writing in 1916)
- Latin names of medicines and chemicals are more distinctive than the vernacular names
- It helps to conceal the kind of medicine being taken and the nature of the disease from the patient themselves (if desirable) and from other 'inquisitive' people who may have more or less legitimate interest in the patient

This is a fascinating historical perspective which has clearly endured to this day though clearly now and in an age of openness and honesty, it is vital, when communicating with children and their families that we ensure that all know what kind of medicine is being given as well as the nature of disease process that is being treated. In theory we do not need to use Latin, though we do continue to do, maybe because of increasing globalisation and the movement of healthcare practitioner from country to country, who all still understand a universal language through their medical education, as well as the fact that it is a space-saving way of writing prescriptions.

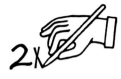

What is a forum?

So far we have discussed the basis of pharmacological practice thus offering a rationale for why we need comprehensive knowledge of pharmacokinetics and dynamics, to looking at the prescription chart and the process of administering medication to children and young people, which now leads us to the calculation process where we need to look in greater depth at the 'right dose' and 'right time' part of the process.

THE NUMBERS – RIGHT DOSE AND RIGHT TIME

The most commonly taught approach to calculating medicine dosages is via use of a formula so this is the starting point for the numerical skills to be developed in this chapter.

What is a formula?

In this context a 'formula' should not be confused with infant 'formula' milk that we give to babies and young children. Within a numerical context it can be defined as a mathematical rule or relationship expressed in symbols or alternatively a set of symbols and numbers that expresses a fact or rule. For example, $A = \pi r^2$ is the formula for calculating the area of a circle or $E = mc^2$ is Einstein's famous formula relating energy and mass.

A formula is a type of equation which shows the relationship between different variables where an equation defines the relationship between two things that are equal, that is, $x + 2 = 5$. The equals sign defines the relationship.

The children's nursing formula contains the variables of amount in mg and mL (or number of capsules, tablets etc.) which can sometimes confuse nurses because we are not using the same units, that is, linking mL and mg when giving medicines in suspension form.

As discussed in Chapter 1 learning a formula can be useful, though it is important to recognise the derivation and understand the principles that underpin it so that the result you get is meaningful and real.

The most common way of calculating amounts of medicines required is by using the formula as follows, though having looked at calculating fractions, percentages, ratios and proportions so far in this book, you will realise there is more than one method that can be used. You also need to be able to calculate using fractions, ratios and proportions to be able to use the formula effectively as well as efficiently. At this stage of the book you can start making decisions around which method works best for you and then solve problems and develop strategies to remember how to do this in practice and in preparation for tests. Have a read through the following, then practice and identify which method works best for you!

The children's nursing formula.

$$\frac{\text{What you want?}}{\text{What you have got?}} \times \frac{\text{What it is in?}}{1} =$$

This is referred to in various ways in different nursing contexts as demonstrated below. Identify the wording that makes more sense to you and use a consistent approach.

Alternative wording.

$$\frac{\text{Strength required}}{\text{Stock strength}} \times \text{Volume of stock solution} =$$

The NHS mnemonic

N = Need (what you want)

H = Have (what you have got)

S = Stock (what it is supplied in or stock strength, usually one table or the volume if in liquid form)

The NHS mnemonic.

$$\frac{\text{N}}{\text{H}} \times \frac{\text{S}}{1} =$$

The following is a worked example using a variety of ways to calculate the amount needed including the formula.

Worked example:

2-year-old Banita from Chapter 2 develops an ear infection and is prescribed an antibiotic, flucloxacillin 250 mg. It is available in a suspension consisting of 125 mg of medicine in 5 mL liquid.

How much will you administer?

Start by estimating what the final amount of suspension should be. The prescribed amount, 250 mg, is bigger than 125 mg (as supplied) so you will need more than 5 mL. The final number must be bigger than 5 mL.

The amount can be calculated in many different ways. What follows are some suggestions:

Method 1: Using mental arithmetic

Some of you at estimation stage will have already identified the amount to be given. Look at the relationship between the numbers involved. How does 250 relate to 125? Can you see that 250 is 2 times bigger than 100? So.... you need twice the amount of liquid, that is, 10 mL.

Method 2: Using proportion

Using proportion notations calculate as follows:

5:125 :: ? : 250   **SO** 5/125 :: ? / 250   **SO** 5/125 × 250 = ?

$$\frac{5 \times 250}{125} = \frac{10 \text{ mL}}{1}$$

OR

We have 125 mg of the medicine in 5 mL solution, which as a ratio is 125:5

We need 250 mg 250 ÷ 125 = 2 × 5 = 10 mL

OR You can set up the problem using a table as follows:

Drug amount in mg	Amount in mL
125	5
250	?

Step 1: Write down the ratio, that is, 125:5

Step 2: Label the numbers in top row of table

Step 3: Put known numbers into the columns

Step 4: Divide the two numbers in the same column, that is, $250 \div 125 = 2$

Step 5: Multiply the answer by the number in the next column, that is, $2 \times 5 = 10$ mL

Method 3: Using the children's nursing formula

$$\frac{\text{What you want} \times \text{What it is in}}{\text{What you have got}} = \text{Amount required}$$

$$\frac{250 \times 5}{125} = 10 \text{ mL}$$

Method 4: Another way could be to work out how much of the suspension is equal to 1 mg

i.e.

$$125 \text{ mg} = 5 \text{ mL so } 1 \text{ mg} = \frac{5}{125}$$

We need 250 mg so we need to multiply 5/125 by $250 = 10$ mL

Following on from this worked example is a whole section of practice examples with useful supporting information included.

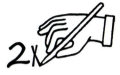

1. **Have a go at the following example that is a bit more complex.**

- Alice is prescribed with some paracetamol 190 mg as an analgesic to treat her headache, as well as for its antipyretic action. The ward stock available is paracetamol 250 mg in 5 mL. Using all the methods outlined above have a go at working out how much will be given to Alice.

APPROVED MEDICINE NAME (PLEASE PRINT)		DATE	03/04			
PARACETAMOL						
DOSE PRN	**ROUTE**	**HOUR**	13			
190 mg	Oral	**MINUTES**	40			
START DATE 03/04/ 2013	**Max. Frequency** 4 - 6 hourly (max 4 doses in 24 hr)	**DOSE GIVEN**	190mg			
SIGNATURE A1Doctor	**BLEEP** 1234	**ROUTE**	Oral			
PRINT NAME A1 Doctor	**PHARMACY** A1P	**SIGN**	ANP/ MEJ			

- It is now 17.15 on the 3 April 2013. Can this dose be given to Alice according to the prescription chart? If yes please sign for it by completing the prescription chart and if not, when can it be given?

2. We can now progress to look at the other medicines prescribed for Alice. Using the same principles and methods calculate the amounts of intravenous antibiotics that need to be given to Alice using the information offered below.

APPROVED MEDICINE NAME (PLEASE PRINT)			**MONTH & DATE**	03/04	04/04	05/04	
CO-AMOXICLAV			Tick or enter variable times				
DOSE	**START DATE**	**ROUTE**	6				
380mg	03.04.2013	IV	12	07.00	X	AN/PT	
			14				
START TIME 15.00	**STOP DATE** 05.04.2013		18	15.00	AN/PT		X
SIGNATURE A1 Doctor		**BLEEP** 1234	22				
PRINT NAME		**PHARMACY**	24	23.00	GJ/LMO		X
A1 DOCTOR		A1 pharmacist					

Whilst it is vitally important to look up these medicines in the BNF whilst in clinical practice, here is some basic information about the antibiotics administered, to keep you focused on the numerical information at hand.

Medicine information: Augmentin injection, tablets, suspension and Augmentin-duo suspension all contain the active ingredients amoxicillin and clavulanic acid, which together are known as co-amoxiclav. Amoxicillin is a penicillin-type antibiotic, and clavulanic acid is a medicine that prevents bacteria from inactivating the amoxicillin. Amoxicillin impairs the bonds that hold the bacterial cell wall together, which allows holes to appear in the cell walls and kills the bacteria. Certain bacteria are resistant to penicillin-type antibiotics, because they have developed the ability to produce defensive chemicals called beta-lactamases. These interfere with the structure of penicillin-type antibiotics and stop them from working whereby clavulanic acid is a type of medicine known as a beta-lactamase inhibitor. It prevents these bacteria from inactivating the amoxicillin, and leaves the bacteria susceptible to attack. Co-amoxiclav is a broad-spectrum antibiotic that kills a wide variety of bacteria that cause a wide variety of commonly occurring infections such as the causative agent of Alice's chest infection, which is not known on admission. It is usually reserved for treating infections caused by bacteria that are resistant to amoxicillin.

Dosage: 30 mg/kg given every 8 hours

Reconstitution advice: 600 mg vial reconstituted with 9.5 mL water for injections gets a final volume of 10 mL

- How much will you give to Alice to get a dose, as prescribed?
- Is this the correct dose based on her weight of 12.6 kg?

Alice develops a rash following administration of the third dose of co-amoxiclav and so the antibiotic is changed to cefotaxime.

APPROVED MEDICINE NAME (PLEASE PRINT)			MONTH & DATE	04/04	05/04	06/04	
Cefotaxime			Tick or enter variable times				
DOSE 630 mg	**START DATE** 03.04.2013	**ROUTE** IV	6				
			12	07.00	X	AN/PT	
			14				
START TIME 15.00	**STOP DATE** 05.04.2013		18				
SIGNATURE Al Doctor		**BLEEP** 1234	22				
PRINT NAME AI DOCTOR		**PHARMACY** SA pharmacist	24	23.00	GJ/2640		X

Medicine information: Cefotaxime is a type of antibiotic called a cephalosporin. These antibiotics are related to penicillin and work in a similar way to co-amoxiclav. Cefotaxime is used to treat infections caused by bacteria and works by interfering with the ability of bacteria to form cell walls. The cell walls of bacteria are vital for their survival. They keep unwanted substances from entering their cells and stop the contents of their cells from leaking out. Cefotaxime impairs the bonds that hold the bacterial cell wall together. As previously this allows holes to appear in the cell walls and kills the bacteria. Cefotaxime is a broad-spectrum antibiotic that kills a wide variety of bacteria that cause a wide variety of commonly occurring infections.

Dose: 50 mg/kg given 12 hourly

Reconstitution: Add 10 mL of diluent to 1 g vial to get 10.4 mL = 95 mg/mL

- How much will you give to Alice to get a dose as prescribed rounded up to one decimal place?
- Is this the correct dose based on her weight of 12.6 kg?

3. Choosing the correct syringe for the job.

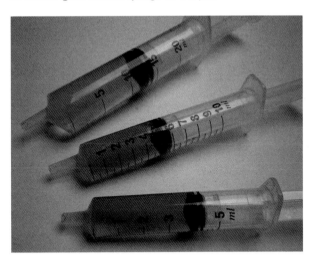

- 5 mL syringe – graduations of 0.2 mL so can give to the nearest 0.2 mL with accuracy
- 10 mL graduations of 0.5 mL so can only administer to the 0.5 mL with accuracy
- 20 mL syringe graduated to the 1 mL so can give only to 1 mL with accuracy

What degree of accuracy can you get when using the syringes pictured?

- Can you give accurate doses of the antibiotics prescribed above? What do you do if you cannot?
- If you give a dose of 625 mg of cefotaxime, does this make the dose easier to measure and give?

4. For Luke's pain to be managed effectively we need to assess his pain using the Arch Mede Pain Assessment tool and then administer analgesics based on his score and our visual assessment of behaviour, following discussion with his parents. We then assess the effectiveness of analgesia given and monitor for any side effects. Non-pharmacological methods should also be considered, that is, ensuring that his arm is placed in a comfortable position and that he feels safe and secure in the ward environment.

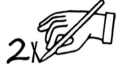

The following table contains a range of analgesics, with some information included and some not. Please fill in the blanks and calculate how much should be prescribed and the dose that should be administered to Luke, if it is the medicine of choice. Clearly not all these analgesics will be given to Luke, who has paracetamol and ibuprofen prescribed on his chart.

Analgesic	Action	Dose	How much for Luke?	Dose supplied in	Dose given
Paracetamol	Non-opioid, analgesic commonly used in children's nursing practice to treat mild to moderate pain and pyrexia	20 mg/kg for severe pain for 48 hours only		250 mg in 5 mL	
Ibuprofen	Non-steroidal anti-inflammatory analgesic for mild to moderate pain	30 mg/kg in 3–4 divided doses		100 mg in 5 mL suspension	
Diclofenac sodium		0.5–1 mg/kg (max 50 mg) 3 times daily	Calculate a 0.5 mg/kg dose =	25 mg/50 mg dispersible tablets	
Codeine phosphate		0.5–1 mg/ kg every 4–6 hours (max 240 mg daily)	Calculate a 0.75 mg/ kg dose =	25 mg in 5 mL	
Morphine		200–500 micrograms/ kg (max 20 mg) every 4 hours titrated to response	Calculate a 300 microgram/ kg dose =	Oral solution supplied in 10 mg/5 mL Note – if the solution is above 13 mg/5 mL it becomes a CD	

Intranasal morphine was given in A&E in a dose of 0.2 mL. This has been stated as a volume (rather than amount in milligrams), which should not be given because there is no amount of morphine specified. This is how it has been calculated as per guidelines used in Arch Mede Hospital A&E department (which are based on guidelines from other A&E departments around the United Kingdom and BNF for children).

The way recommended is to weigh the child to the nearest 5 kg and round down using the table below. Dilute 10 mg of diamorphine with the specific volume of sterile water as indicated and then draw up 0.2 mL which will give the child a dose of 100 microgram/kg (or 0.1 mg/kg in 0.2 mL).

Child's weight (in kg)	Volume of sterile water (in mL) added to a 10 mg ampoule	Dose of diamorphine (in mg)
10	2	1
15	1.3	1.5
20	1	2
25	0.8	2.5
30	0.7	2.86
35	0.6	3.33
40	0.5	4
45	0.45	4.44
50	0.4	5

Can you see the pattern of numbers in the table where the smaller the child the greater the amount of diluent added to get the required concentration. You can probably see how errors could occur and as a result see why medicines should be prescribed in milligrams and not millilitres if supplied in milligrams.

In addition to completing the activities you could look up the medicines identified in the BNF for children to find out what they are and why they are used in children's nursing.

- What are the usual dosages and what are the side effects that you may need to inform parents and young people about?
- Is there anything else you need to think about when administering medicines to children as compared with adults?

Safety hints and tips: Remember to sign the prescription chart using initials immediately after a medicine is given and be aware of the side effects and observe for them following administration.

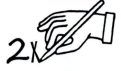

Examples of range of typical medications used in children's nursing practice. There are more examples for practice purposes on the ONE resource.

Weight (if needed)	Medicine	Amount	Route	Frequency	Numeracy problem to be solved	Answer
	Chlorpheniramine	1 mg	Oral	t.d.s.	Supplied in an oral liquid 2 mg in 5 mL. How much will you give?	
	Diazepam	2.5 mg	Oral	Single dose	Supplied in an oral liquid 2 mg in 5 mL. How much will you give?	
13.5 kg	Alfacalcidol	400 nanograms	Oral	Daily	2 micrograms per mL	
12 kg	Cefalexin	30 mg/kg/day	Oral	q.d.s.	Calculate the single does to be given	

Weight (if needed)	Medicine	Amount	Route	Frequency	Numeracy problem to be solved	Answer
36 kg	Flucloxacillin	100 mg/ kg/day	Oral	q.d.s.	Calculate the single does to be given	
	Amoxicillin	160 mg	IV	t.d.s.	The antibiotic is made up so that you have 100 mg/mL. How much will be given?	
	Amoxicillin	160 mg	IV	t.d.s.	The antibiotic is made up so that you have 250 mg/mL. How much will be given?	

CONCLUDING COMMENTS

This chapter has focused in on the use of a formula as well as other methods to calculate medicine dosages for children and young people using the experiences of two children – Alice and Luke, who were admitted for very different reasons, thus allowing a range of medicines to serve as a basis for the calculations that support this chapter . These numeracy skills have been set within the context of the medicine administration process in children focusing in on the special needs relating to young children in particular. In the next chapter we will follow a similar theme though will add a level of complexity to the calculations thus supporting the care of the neonate and much younger children in a critical care/high-dependency environment as a result.

Chapter 6

. . . .

ADMINISTERING MEDICINES AND MANAGING NUMBERS IN MORE COMPLEX SETTINGS – THE PHARMACIST AND NEONATAL NURSING PERSPECTIVES

Gerard Donaghy and Lisa Mccormack

Numeracy in Children's Nursing, First Edition. Arija Parker
© 2015 John Wiley & Sons, Ltd. Published 2015 by John Wiley & Sons Ltd.

LEARNING FOCUS

The focus will be on the experiences of a neonate and the numbers that relate to his/her care thus emphasising the added complexities and dependence on numerical ability in high dependency and critical care settings in children and young people's practice.

LEARNING OBJECTIVES

By the end of this chapter you should be able to:

- Develop your skills in calculating medication dosages and fluid calculations to a higher level
- Increase your knowledge of care of infants, children and young people in high dependency/intensive care settings
- Appreciate the importance of multidisciplinary working when using numbers in practice – the common understanding and interpretation of prescription charts in our practice

CASE SCENARIO 8

Robert (called Bobby for short) has been admitted to Alpha Ward 1 (the Neonatal Intensive Care Unit) at Arch Mede Hospital. His mum was admitted yesterday following a routine antenatal appointment where it was noticed that the baby had reduced foetal movements. At the time his mum, Ms. Babbage, was 31 weeks into her pregnancy, where until 29 weeks, she had an uneventful pregnancy. She presented with spontaneous rupture of membranes and received two doses of steroids 24 hours apart and was discharged home with a follow-up in 2 weeks.

The reason for administering antenatal steroids is because they are associated with a significant reduction in rates of neonatal death, respiratory distress syndrome and intraventricular haemorrhage (RCOG, 2010).

Hospital number	AMH2014-08
Ward	Alpha Ward 1 (NICU)
Weight	1.35 kg (Between 9th and 25th centile)

Baseline observations.

Temperature	Pulse	Blood pressure	Respirations	CRT	Pain score	Blood sugar
36.7° C	140 bpm	26 mmHg (mean)	49 per minute (via ventilator)	<3 seconds	2	2.3 mmol/L

Blood results for Bobby on admission to Alpha Ward 1.

Urea and electrolytes		Normal ranges for neonate	Full blood count		Normal ranges for neonate
Sodium	142	133–146 mmol/L	Haemoglobin	16.5	12.5–20.5 g/dL
Potassium	5.3	3.5–5.3 mmol/L	White cell count	11.9	5–20 × 10⁹/L
Urea	6.2	2.5–7.8 mmol/L	Platelets	215	140–440 × 10⁹/L
Creatinine	75	21–75 mmol/L			
CRP	23	0–5 mg/L			

Bobby was commenced on a heparin infusion to be infused into his umbilical arterial catheter (UAC). The infusion is set to be infused at 0.5 mL/hr at a concentration of 0.5 units/mL in sodium chloride 0.45% to be infused into his umbilical arterial catheter. He was also commenced on an infusion of morphine at 10 micrograms/kg/hr. This is to provide pain relief and a moderate form of sedation which is required when babies are on a ventilator.

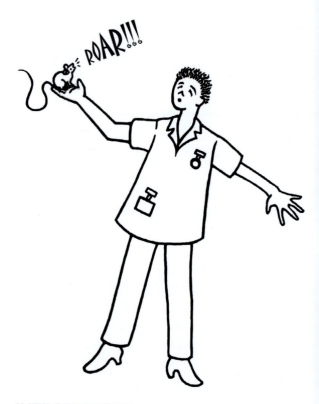

INTRODUCTION

Just as you are now improving your confidence and competence with use of numbers and probably starting to feel more comfortable with these skills it is time to push you out of this comfort zone. This chapter will help us look at how calculations play an important part in practice and how they are used, prescribed and administered in the care of babies on a Neonatal Intensive Care Unit. We will look at how medication is prescribed and the mathematics behind that, the various forms of medication that a nurse will come across in this field, and how this medication is prepared and administered to very small babies. Often medications are supplied in larger denominations than those prescribed, necessitating conversions to be made in either the prescribing, preparation or drawing up stages prior to administration.

Incorrect conversions can result in errors to a factor of ten or more. Neonatal Intensive Care nurses therefore need to be able to accurately convert and calculate medication dosages. Bobby's experiences will guide the discussion where issues arising will be explained and numerical data expanded on as worked examples. The role of the hospital pharmacist will also be considered within these discussions and around Bobby's hospital care.

At the start of each section, where relating numbers to Bobby's care there will be a question asking you to have a go at answering the question before moving on to look at the worked example. Also have a think about alternative ways of doing the calculations based on the skills developed in earlier chapters.

Why are children and neonates different?

Children are not mini adults

Although the way in which children handle medication is basically the same, this is not always the case. Some of the mechanisms by which children absorb and metabolise medication take time to develop and mature, and this process can take possibly weeks or months to occur. There are also changes in the way that children distribute and excrete medicines. These factors should be considered when looking at the appropriateness of medication use in children and neonates.

Before we focus in on these areas of practice let us continue the story of Bobby – he was born by normal vaginal delivery weighing 1.35 kg and at birth his APGAR scores are: 6, 8 and 8. He began grunting at 5 minutes after birth , became tachypnoeic and required oxygen to maintain oxygen saturations above 88%.

The Apgar Score

The Apgar score was developed in 1952 by the American anesthetist Dr. Virginia Apgar as an easy and repeatable method to quickly assess the health of newborn children immediately after birth.

The Apgar score is determined by evaluating the newborn baby on five simple criteria on a scale from 0 to 2 through simple addition of the categories. The resulting Apgar score ranges from 0 to 10. The five criteria are summarised using words chosen to form an acronym (Appearance, Pulse, Grimace, Activity, Respiration). It is quick, simple and easy to use.

Clinical feature	Score			Acronym
	0	1	2	
Colour of trunk	White or Blue	Pink with blue extremities	Pink	Appearance
Heart rate	0	≤100	>100	Pulse
Response to pharyngeal catheter	Nil	Grimace	Cough	Grimace
Muscle tone	Limp	Diminished, or normal with no movements	Normal with active movements	Activity
Respiration	Absent	Gasping or irregular	Regular or crying lustily	Respiration

Source: Rennie (Ed) (2005)

Bobby was placed in the transport incubator and transferred from delivery suite to the neonatal unit aged 12 minutes. On admission, his temperature was taken. Blood samples were taken for: a blood culture, full blood count and DCT, C-reactive protein, blood group and save, blood gas, blood glucose and first day blood spot. He received a 400 microgram/kg dose of Vitamin K (phytomenadione) by IM injection. The reason for this is to help prevent the baby from developing haemorrhagic disease of the newborn. Bobby was commenced on 60 mL/kg/day of 10% glucose following a capillary blood glucose level of 3.2 mmol/L.

Bobby was commenced on first-line antibiotics of benzylpenicillin and gentamicin during his admission to cover against the risk of the common early onset neonatal infections of Group B *Streptococci* and *Escherichia Coli*. He was commenced on a form of non-invasive ventilation known as nasal continuous positive airway pressure (nCPAP), following an infusion of caffeine citrate at 20 mg/kg over 20 minutes.

His blood gases were checked after 1 hour, and were deemed to be satisfactory. He had an X-ray at 4 hours of age, which showed a bilateral ground glass appearance, which is mostly likely attributed to surfactant deficient lung disease or infection. He was intubated at 5 hours of age, following a dose of 100 micrograms/kg of morphine and suxamethonium of 2 mg/kg, and the surfactant poractant alfa was administered via endotracheal tube. The reason for this was due to increased oxygen requirements and worsening blood gas results and X-ray findings.

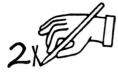

What is Surfactant?

Surfactant is a mixture of substances including phospholipids, neutral lipids and proteins. Its main function is to reduce the surface tension in the lungs and to help open alveoli. It does this by sticking to the side of the airways and gives them more stability in expiration. It also prevents the process of transudation, where fluid is sucked back into the alveoli from the capillaries in instances of high surface tension within the lung.

The Advanced Neonatal Nursing Practitioner (ANNP) inserted umbilical venous and arterial catheters. This is to allow arterial blood to be sampled from an inline device and reduce painful procedures in the neonate. Arterial catheters also enable blood pressure monitoring which is considered to be more accurate than using a cuff. The venous catheter is used for administration of IV fluids and drug infusions.

His observations and bloods were rechecked and the baseline results are given above.

Bobby, the nurse and the pharmacist

- **The role of the hospital pharmacist**

Hospital pharmacists are experts in the field of medicines. They work closely with medical and nursing staff to ensure patients receive the most appropriate treatment, and provide help and advice to patients in all aspects of their medicines.

They advise on the selection of medicines, the dose, preparation and route of administration for individual patients. They provide information about potential side effects and ensure that new treatments are compatible with existing medication in terms of physical and clinical interactions. In addition, they monitor the effects of treatment to ensure that it is safe and effective.

Pharmacists have a responsibility to follow their standards of conduct, ethics and performance as issued by the General Pharmaceutical Council. There are seven principles to follow and they revolve around the patient and those they work with. They are:

1. Make patients your first concern
2. Use your professional judgement in the interest of patients and the public
3. Show respect for others
4. Encourage patients and the public to participate in decisions about their care
5. Develop your professional knowledge and competence
6. Be honest and trustworthy
7. Take responsibility for your working practices

The General Medical Council has issued guidance with regards to prescribing of medication in 2008. It is a guide to situations that doctors may find themselves in relation to their practice.

The main principles are:

- Keeping up to date and prescribing in patients' best interests
- Keeping patients' general practitioners informed
- Doctors' interests in pharmacies
- Prescribing situations requiring special consideration
- Prescribing controlled drugs for yourself or someone close to you
- Prescribing for patients to whom you also dispense
- Prescribing unlicensed medicines

- Prescribing medicines for use outside the terms of their license (off-label)
- Information for patients about the license for their medicines
- Responsibility for prescribing medicines for hospital outpatients

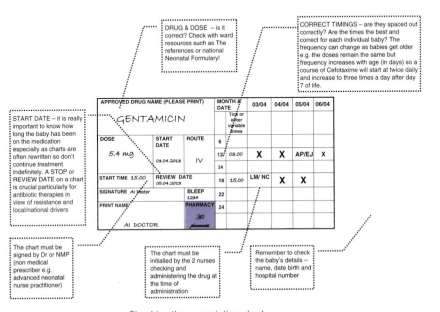

DRUG & DOSE – is it correct? Check with ward resources such as The references or national Neonatal Formulary!

CORRECT TIMINGS – are they spaced out correctly? Are the times the best and correct for each individual baby? The frequency can change as babies get older e.g. the doses remain the same but frequency increases with age (in days) so a course of Cefotaxime will start at twice daily and increase to three times a day after day 7 of life.

START DATE – it is really important to know how long the baby has been on the medication especially as charts are often rewritten so don't continue treatment indefinitely. A STOP or REVIEW DATE on a chart is crucial particularly for antibiotic therapies in view of resistance and local/national drivers

The chart must be signed by Dr or NMP (non medical prescriber e.g. advanced neonatal nurse practitioner)

The chart must be initialled by the 2 nurses checking and administering the drug at the time of administration

Remember to check the baby's details – name, date birth and hospital number

Checking the prescription chart.

• The role of the nurse

Nurses are accountable for their own practice with regards to drug administration. It is not a defence of action or error to simply administer a drug which has been prescribed. The nurse must be knowledgeable with regard to indications for use, side effects, dosing, preparation and administration – it is not acceptable to administer a drug because 'the doctor prescribed it' as prescribing errors can be made and the nurse is usually the professional responsible for administering it. Therefore the nurse needs to take responsibility to familiarise themselves with the drugs used, doses and so on for any area/ward they work in.

'The administration of medicines is an important aspect of the professional practice of persons whose names are on the Council's register. It is not solely a mechanistic task to be performed in strict compliance with the written prescription of a medical practitioner (can now also be an independent and supplementary prescriber). It requires thought and the exercise of professional judgement...' (NMC, 2010).

Why mistakes happen revisited with emphasis on the neonatal perspective

The issues of mistakes and error have been discussed in the early chapters of this book and now need revisiting and reiterating in general and with a focus on the neonate. A medication error can be described as any error in the prescribing, dispensing or administration of a medication. Medication errors may be classified according to the stage of the medication use cycle in which they occur (prescribing, dispensing or administration). Incidences of medication error rates vary widely, dependent on the reporting system used and whether they are reported appropriately or not. The majority of medication errors occur as a result of poor prescribing and often involve relatively inexperienced medical staff who are responsible for the majority of prescribing in hospital (Williams, 2007).

Errors can be attributed to three categories:

* Prescribing errors
* Dispensing errors
* Administration errors

A prescribing error can be defined as an incorrect drug selection for a patient. These errors can include the dose, frequency, name or prescribing of a contraindicated drug.

Other factors that can be construed as prescribing errors include:

* Illegible handwriting.
* Inaccurate medication transcription from GP list or patient's own medication.
* Confusion with the drug name, for example, amiloride and amlodipine.

- Inappropriate use of decimal points. A zero should always precede a decimal point (e.g. 0·1 not .1). Similarly, 10-fold errors in dose have occurred as a result of the use of a trailing zero (e.g. 1 should never be written as 1·0).
- Use of abbreviations (e.g. mcg being misinterpreted as mg and the use of U to define units which if written badly may be mistaken for a 0).

Approaches to reducing dispensing errors include:

- Ensuring safe dispensing procedures are in place separating drugs with a similar name or those that are in similar packaging both in pharmacy and on the ward area when drugs are being selected.
- Keeping interruptions in the dispensing procedure to a minimum and maintaining the workload of the pharmacist at a safe and manageable level.
- Awareness of high-risk drugs such as potassium chloride and controlled drugs.

Some approaches to try to reduce drug administration errors include:

- Checking the patient's identity by more than one healthcare professional.
- Ensuring that dosage calculations are checked independently by another healthcare professional before the drug is administered using recognised reference sources where appropriate.
- Ensuring that the prescription, drug, and patient are in the same place in order that they may be checked against one another.
- Ensuring the medication is given at the correct time.
- Minimising interruptions during drug rounds.
- Ensuring that errors are reported in a timely manner, so that problems and trends can be identified and training put in place to rectify if necessary.

An example of this is gentamicin, an antibiotic used 'routinely' on the neonatal unit as a first-line treatment for proven or suspected infection. It is prescribed for Bobby as a 24 or 36 hourly drug depending upon the gestation of the baby and thus the ability of the body to deal with its excretion (see the chart above for Bobby's prescription of gentamicin). However, as gentamicin is always prescribed alongside another antibiotic to provide a broad spectrum of cover against various infections, it has often been given too early as the antibiotic that is prescribed alongside is a 12 hourly/twice daily required drug. Thus the nurse has given both antibiotics at the same time every time. The nature of potential harm or side effect caused by an overdose of gentamicin namely hearing loss and renal damage is so great that in 2010 the National Patient Safety Agency (NPSA) issued guidance and a pre-administration checklist to act as a prompt and reduce the administration errors of gentamicin following 507 patient safety incidents between April 2008 and March 2009 in neonates. This is just the number of incidences reported, it may be a far greater number as errors are not always reported or discovered. However 96% of these incidents reported no/low harm but 23 babies suffered moderate harm as a result of gentamicin.

The latest prescribing advice can be found at https://www.nice.org.uk/guidance/cg149 where all prescribing of Gentamicin should be 5 mg/kg every 36 hours, which was not the guidance that was available when Bobby was born.

So how can errors be prevented? Obviously no one sets out to intentionally cause harm but when working with small, immature babies whose ability to deal with a drug may be less than an older child or adult, the margin for error is minute and should of course be non-existent. But we are human and mistakes can happen – working in a busy, noisy and stressful environment can affect concentration on the task of medication administration – alarms on babies sounding or parents but more often than not other colleagues! Strategies to reduce interruptions have nationally included the wearing of a red tabard during drug rounds to alert others to the fact that drugs are being prepared. However, as neonatal units do not tend to have drug rounds due to the frequency of drugs being required a red tabard would need to be worn almost constantly and thus reduce the visual impact of it! Other concerns about these have included infection control.

Clinical pharmacists are key to ensuring the safe use of medicines and pharmacists visiting wards or being based on wards place them in a good position to recognise particular training needs and can proactively assist in implementing good practice and delivering training to those that require it.

Off-label/not licensed for neonatal use

The vast majority of medications that are used in newborn babies are licensed. However there are instances that children are required to take medication that is either unlicensed or off-label. These are often needed when there is a lack of suitable licensed medication for use in children and, consequently, a lack of appropriate formulations that children can take in suitable volumes. The main reason for the use of these medications in children is a lack of clinical trials due to the significant cost of them.

Neonatal Nursing perspectives

Babies often on multiple drug regimens and timing is important to ensure serum drug levels are maintained – neonatal units do not have 'drug rounds' whereby patients have drugs at set times as can historically happen in a more task-orientated environment. Drugs are often rewritten if doses are late because of IV access problems so keeping check on what is due can be tricky if at first glance a chart has multiple crossings out. The neonatal nurse may have to ask the doctor/NMP to re-prescribe all of the drugs on to a new chart to ensure it is clear what is due. Babies on multiple drugs/infusions may even have two charts in use which again can be a risk as omissions can occur.

The small doses prescribed/required make it easy to miscalculate especially in an emergency situation. Neonatal medications are usually prescribed in milligrams or micrograms but the supply may be a higher denomination requiring conversion to take place so that the calculation involves numbers in the same units.

Fill in the blanks in the table below

SI conversions

Kilogram (kg)	Gram (g)	Milligram (mg)	Microgram	Nanogram
0.001	1	1000	1000000	1000000000
		6		
	800			
			20	
				250000
2.75				

Drug reconstitution can be complex, for example, vancomycin which requires reconstitution then further dilution to make it a more manageable volume to give over the required time, that is, an hour. Interruptions by other staff and/or parents and baby monitors alarming add an extra dimension to what is already a complex task.

Look back at the Six Rights in Chapter 5 –does this approach need to be modified for neonates?

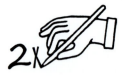

The etiquette of prescribing using BNF for children

1. The unnecessary use of decimal points should be avoided – is 3.0 mg correct?
2. Quantities of 1 gram or more should be written as 1 g – so if 1500 mg is prescribed how should it be written?
3. Quantities less than 1 gram should be written in milligrams, that is, 0.5 g =
4. Quantities less than 1 mg should be written in micrograms, that is, 0.75 mg =

5. When decimals are unavoidable a zero should be written in front of the decimal point where there is no other figure, that is, is .5 mg correct? How should it be written?

6. Use of the decimal point is acceptable to express a range, for example, 0.5– 1 g. TRUE OR FALSE?

7. 'Micrograms' and 'nanograms' should **not** be abbreviated. Similarly 'units' should **not** be abbreviated. TRUE OR FALSE?

8. The term 'millilitre' (mL) is used in medicine and pharmacy, and cubic centimetre, c.c., or cm³ should not be used. TRUE OR FALSE?

Source: BNF for Children (2011–2012)

The practicalities of caring and making nursing decisions for a neonate – the focus on numbers

When a shift commences it is good and safe practice to check all infusions and fluids to ensure they are running at the correct rate. Going back to basics, the easiest way to do this is to start with what the total fluid requirement is for the day: this is a medical decision based on the overall clinical condition of the baby and gestation. Once you know how much fluid is required you can check the hourly rate; this is the total requirement for the day divided by 24 (hours). You then go to your prescription chart, fluid chart and pumps and look at what drugs are running at a prescribed rate to give a certain dose. You must subtract all of the prescribed drug rates from this hourly rate to then leave you with the rate at which the maintenance fluid should be running at.

So, taking our patient Bobby, if his total daily fluid requirement is 90 mL/Kg or 90 millilitres per kilogram of weight – he weighs 1.35 kg so you multiply this by 90.

$90 \times 1.35 = 121.5$ mL

So divide this by 24 to work out how much fluid is required every hour = 5.06 mL.

We can have a total of 5.06 mL

0.15 mL of morphine + 0.5 mL of heparin = 0.65 mL

5.06 − 0.65 = 4.41 mL maintenance fluid per hour.

Maintenance fluid

This will provide sufficient fluid for hydration and glucose for energy. The first choice of fluid is glucose 10%. By 72 hours of age when diuresis has occurred, the requirements alter so that sodium supplementation is necessary – glucose10% with sodium chloride 0.18% is an option used but NICU polices on this may vary. Total parenteral nutrition (TPN) may also be required depending on how Bobby progresses with his feeds.

Dilution fluid

The choice of diluent (the fluid used to dilute medications) depends on both the properties of the drug, that is, what it is stable in but also the condition of the baby. High or low sodium levels in the blood, or glucose may influence the clinicians choice. This sometimes requires the nurse to remake infusions as the critically ill baby is very fine to balance with slight changes making a big difference to their overall condition.

When babies are very small it is sometimes necessary to double or even quadruple the strength of a drug infusion as a standard strength would mean too large a volume infusing especially if many drugs are required. A tiny 23-week gestation baby weighing 500 g (0.5 Kg) and on a fluid requirement of 120 mL/Kg/day = 60 mL – if they were requiring dopamine, dobutamine, morphine, parental nutrition, lipid, insulin, heparinised saline, adrenaline is expected to have all this delivered in just 2.5 mL every hour! You can see why concentrating the infusion would be necessary but absolutely crucial to get it right.

Focus in on neonatal practice in your own hospital. How do you work out whether the infusion is running at the correct rate?

When in your own unit you can refer to your local pharmacopoeia but if you go to work at another unit or is involved in the transport of babies you may come across different strengths and ways of making up infusions. One method to calculate whether the rate is correct is as follows:

Check the prescription to see how much drug has been prescribed.

Divide by the volume it has been made up in – this gives you how many milligrams in 1 mL (if working in micrograms multiply by 1000).

Divide subtotal by the baby's weight (if working in a drug prescribed per minute divide by 60).

Times by the rate = what it is running at (dose).

PHYSIOLOGY AND NUMERACY RELATED TO BOBBY

Intravenous medication – the theory

So let us use the case study to explore the numbers that relate to Bobby by exploring why calculating intravenous medication is so important and how to analyse the data we are presented with by observing Bobby, measuring vital signs and looking at laboratory results.

In children water forms 45–75% of total body weight. An infant has the highest amount of water per body weight, that is, premature infant at 90%, newborn infant at 70–80% and at 1–2 years old 64%.

Total body water has a significant role in the dosing of medication in children, especially those who are born prematurely.

Such changes in body composition can affect the apparent volume of distribution of a drug. For example, gentamicin is distributed in total body water and has greater volumes of distribution in neonates and infants. As a result of this doses generally need to be increased.

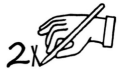

What dose of benzylpenicillin would you expect Bobby to be prescribed if he was born weighing 1.35 kg. The dose of benzylpenicillin is 25 mg/kg twice a day.

What dose of gentamicin would you expect Bobby to be prescribed at 5 mg/kg every 36 hours?

Displacement values defined

A displacement value is the volume occupied by the powder when a suitable diluent is added during reconstitution. This is particularly important to take into account when the dose needed is only a proportion of the vial content.

If we look at benzylpenicillin injection as an example:

The displacement volume for benzylpenicillin 600 mg is 0.4 mL. Therefore if 5.6 mL of diluent is added to a 600 mg vial, the resulting solution is benzylpenicillin 600 mg in 6 mL.

Note: The displacement volume is different for each drug, for each strength of drug and for different brands/ manufacturers' formulae.

The usual ones used at Arch Mede Hospital are as follows:

Co-amoxiclav 600 mg has a displacement value of 0.5 mL. We add 9.5 mL to get a concentration of 60 mg per mL.

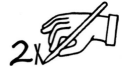

How much diluent do we need to add to the following examples?

Amoxicillin 500 mg in a final volume of 5 mL has a displacement value of 0.4 mL.

Flucloxacillin 250 mg in a final volume of 2.5 mL has a displacement value of 0.2 mL.

Vancomycin 500 mg in a final volume of 10 mL has a displacement value of 0.3 mL.

Meropenem 500 mg in a final volume of 5 mL has a displacement value of 0.5 mL.

Cefotaxime 500 mg in a final of 5 mL has a displacement value of 0.2 mL.

Calculating fluid requirements in neonates

	Term	Preterm	<1000 g	IUGR
Day 1	60	60	90	90
Day 2	90	90	120	120
Day 3	120	120	120	150
Day 4	150	120	150	180
Day 5 and on	150	150/200	150	

Fluid balance is crucial in the intensive care environment so the neonatal nurse must carefully chart all fluid going into and out of the baby. The input is easier as it includes infusions at set rates, flushes, boluses, drugs, blood products or feeds. The output is a bit more difficult. Whilst it is easy enough to measure how much blood may be withdrawn to sample or to weigh a nappy, the neonate is subject to insensible water losses through the skin and respiratory tract. For this reason all inspired gases whether this is via the ventilator, nasal CPAP or high-flow device are warmed and humidified. Neonates are also nursed in incubators with the facility to humidify their environment. A 24–25 week baby in 50% humidity can lose up to 140 mL/Kg/day through transepidermal water loss in the first 1–2 days of life; 100 mL/Kg at day 5 and around 50 mL/kg/day at day 28 (Modi, 2004). Water loss occurs as a result of thin, immature skin with a relatively high body surface area to weight. After birth, the skin will keratinise which acts as a barrier to water loss. However careful nursing care is required to minimise this water loss and monitor temperature.

Urine output is another critical measurement in the intensive care environment as it gives an indication as to how well the baby is. Measuring urine output is an approximate science: weight of full nappy – (minus) weight of dry nappy = total. You then divide this by the number of hours since last nappy change (in intensive care this could be up to 12-hourly because of minimal handling principles) divided by the babies' weight to give mL/kg/hour. This gives an idea of how well, or not, the kidneys are working – leaky immature kidneys, output can exceed input – electrolyte imbalance. The urine output of a neonate should be 2–4 mL/kg/hour; <1 mL/kg/hour requires investigation; >6–7 mL/kg/hour suggests excess fluid administration or an impaired concentrating ability (Modi, 2004). Total input and output are required to give a full clinical picture of the baby, and hourly accumulative totals can give an immediate or evolving picture of the condition.

Have a look at Bobby's fluid balance chart in Section 1 for further details

Fluid management – building on previous knowledge

As Bobby was 1.35 kg, he was commenced on 60 mL/kg/day of glucose 10%

- What rate should this infusion be infused at, given the infusions that are also prescribed?

So 60 mL × 1.35 = 81 mL in 24 hours.

So per hour = 81

24 = 3.375 mL/hr but rounded to 3.37 due to the pump only running at two decimal places.
Bobby was commenced on a heparin infusion to be infused into his UAC. The infusion is set to be infused at 0.5 mL/hr at a concentration of 0.25 units/mL in sodium chloride 0.45%.

- What is the most convenient way to make up this solution?

Heparin sodium is supplied in 1000 unit/mL.

Sodium chloride 0.45% comes in 500 mL.

Take 0.25 mL of solution from the 500 mL bag of sodium chloride 0.45% and add 0.25 mL of heparin 1000 units/mL to the bag. This gives a solution of 250 units in 500 mL of sodium chloride 0.45%.

Withdraw 50 mL of this solution into a syringe and infuse at 0.5 mL/hr.

Expanding our knowledge of SI Units: Introduction to moles and millimoles

The mole is a unit of measurement used in chemistry to express amounts of a chemical substance defined as an amount of a substance that contains as many elementary entities as there are atoms in 12 grams of pure carbon-12 (12 C), the isotope of carbon with atomic weight 12. This corresponds to a value of $6.02214179(30) \times 10^{23}$ elementary entities of the substance.

The number of molecules in a mole (known as Avogadro's number) is defined such that the mass of one mole of a substance, expressed in grams, is exactly equal to the substance's mean molecular weight. For example, the mean molecular weight of natural water is about 18.015, so one mole of water is about 18.015 grams. This property considerably simplifies many chemical and physical computations.

So to illustrate this in relation to Bobby we need to work out how many millimoles of sodium is Bobby getting per kilogram of body weight from this infusion?

From the basic chemistry number of mmols = Mass (mg)

Molecular Weight

So let us work out the mass (in grams) of sodium chloride in 500 mL of 0.45% solution.

So 0.45% means 0.45 g in 100 mL.

To convert grams to milligrams so as to remove decimal places we have to multiply by 1000.

So: 0.45 g × 1000 = 450 mg in 100 mL of solution.

Therefore in 1000 mL there will be 450 × 10 = 4500 mg.

To work out the formula mass of sodium chloride we need to use the Periodic Table of Elements.

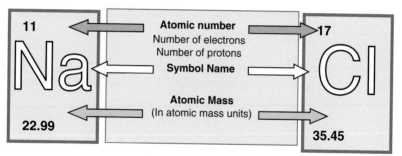

Information about Sodium and Chlorine taken from the periodic table of elements so that you can see where the information for the calculation comes from.

The Periodic table can be accessed at: http://quizlet .com/10651712/nursing-basic-chem-flash-cards

Molecular weight of sodium per mole = 23

Molecular weight of chlorine per mole = 35.5

Therefore the combined molecular weight per mole is 58.5

Therefore the number of mmol = 4500 mg

58.5 = 77mmol in 1 L of 0.45% sodium chloride

Therefore in 1 mL of solution there will be 0.077 mmol of sodium

Bobby will get 12 mL of heparin in 0.45% sodium chloride as 0.5 mL × 24 = 12 mL

Therefore Bobby will get 0.77 mmol × 12 = 0.924 mmol/day

Therefore Bobby is 1.35 kg so to get the value per kilo of body weight we need to divide 0.924 mmol by 1.35 kg

This gives 0.68 mmol/kg/day

Calculating morphine requirements

Bobby becomes quite agitated on the ventilator and is commenced on an infusion of morphine.

How is a 20 mL infusion of morphine prepared so that 0.1 mL/hr equates to 10 micrograms/kg/hr?

So we know that 0.1 mL = 10 micrograms/kg

Therefore 10 mL = 1000 micrograms/kg

Therefore 20 mL = 2000 micrograms/kg

Therefore 20 mL = 2000 micrograms × 1.35

Therefore 20 mL = 2700 micrograms

So we have to put 2.7 mg in 20 mL so that the infusion is correctly made.

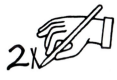

Morphine can come in various strengths from 1 mg/mL, 10 mg/mL, 15 mg/mL, 30 mg/mL and 60 mg/mL. What do you think would be the most appropriate strength to be in the preparation of the infusion and why?

So an alternative formula to make to the infusion

$$\text{Amount of drug (micrograms)} = \frac{\text{Volume in syringe (mL)} \times \text{Dose (microgram/kg/hr)}}{\text{Rate of infusion (mL/hr)}}$$

So in our example above

$$\text{Amount of drug (micrograms)} = \frac{20 \text{ mL} \times 10 \text{ micrograms/hr} \times 1.35 \text{ kg}}{0.1 \text{ mL/hr}}$$

Amount of drug (micrograms) = 2700 micrograms

$$\text{Amount of drug (mg)} = \frac{2700}{1000}$$

$$= 2.7 \text{ mg}$$

However we already know that Bobby is on infusions of heparin at 0.5 mL/hr and morphine at 0.1 mL/hr.

So to calculate the infusion rate to be set:

3.37 − 0.5 − 0.1 = 2.78 mL/hr

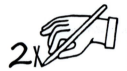

The doctor wants to increase the dose of morphine that Bobby is receiving to 15 micrograms/kg/hr. What would the rate of the infusion have to be changed to?

So assuming that our calculation above is correct, and 0.1 mL/hr equates to 10 micrograms/kg/hr, it would be logical to assume that if the rate of infusion was increased to 0.15 mL/hr then the dose would be increased to 15 micrograms/kg/hr.

However, let us check it to be certain.

$$\text{Amount of drug (micrograms)} = \frac{\text{Volume in syringe (mL)} \times \text{Dose (microgram/kg/hr)}}{\text{Rate of infusion (mL/hr)}}$$

$$2.7 \text{ mg} = 2700 \text{ micrograms}$$

$$2700 \text{ micrograms} = \frac{20 \text{ mL} \times 15 \text{ micrograms/kg/hr}}{\text{Rate of infusion (mL/hr)}}$$

$$\text{Rate of infusion (mL/hr)} = \frac{20 \text{ mL} \times 15 \text{ micrograms/kg/hr}}{2700 \text{ micrograms}}$$

$$\text{Rate of infusion (mL/hr)} = \frac{300 \times 1.35}{2700}$$

$$\text{Rate of infusion (mL/hr)} = 0.15$$

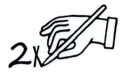

Can you calculate what his total fluid input (in mL/kg) has been over the last 24 hours?

Heparin	24 hours of 0.5 mL/hr
Morphine	6 hours of 0.1 mL/hr
	18 hours of 0.15 mL/hr
Maintenance fluids	6 hours of 2.77 mL/hr
	18 hours of 2.72 mL/hr

After 24 hours Bobby is considered well enough to increase his fluids to 90 mL/kg/day.

At what rate do the maintenance fluids need to be prescribed assuming that the doses of heparin and morphine remain unaltered?

$$\frac{90 \times 1.35}{24} = 5.06 \text{ mL/hr}$$

$$5.06 - 0.5 - 0.15 = 4.41 \text{ mL/hr}$$

Calculating Dopamine requirements

During the day, Bobby's blood pressure drops considerably from a mean of 32 to a mean of 25, as measured from the UAC. The reason for this is thought to be due to the infection. It is decided by the consultant to commence on an infusion of dopamine to help improve his blood pressure following a sodium chloride 0.9% fluid bolus of 10 mL/kg over 30 minutes.

She wants to commence the infusion at 5 micrograms/kg/min which runs at 0.25 mL/hr.

- How is a 50 mL infusion of dopamine prepared so that 0.5 mL/hr equates to 10 micrograms/kg/min?

Dopamine comes as a vial of 200 mg/5 mL.

- So what calculations do we have to carry out in order to work this out?

First of all we need to calculate the amount of dopamine in micrograms that we need in 50 mL.

We can use the formula that we used for the morphine infusion again.

$$\text{Amount of drug (micrograms)} = \frac{\text{Volume in syringe (mL)} \times \text{Dose (microgram/kg/min)}}{\text{Rate of infusion (mL/hr)}}$$

Be careful as the dose is expressed in terms of micrograms/kg/min, but the rate of infusion is in mL/hr. So we need to add in a multiplication of 60 to convert the dose into micrograms/kg/hr.

So we know:

The volume of syringe = 50 mL

The dose = 10 micrograms/kg/min

The rate = 0.5 mL/hr.

So let us put these into our formula

$$\textbf{Amount of drug (micrograms)} = \frac{\textbf{50 mL} \times \textbf{10 micrograms/kg/min}}{\textbf{0.5 mL/hr}}$$

Remember we have to multiply by 60 to convert our dose to hours

$$\textbf{Amount of drug (micrograms)} = \frac{\textbf{50 mL} \times \textbf{10 micrograms} \times \textbf{1.35} \times \textbf{60}}{\textbf{0.5 mL/hr}}$$

Amount of drug (micrograms) = 81000 micrograms

So to convert to milligram divide by 1000 = 81 mg

- So we know that we need 81 mg, and we know that the solution comes in 200 mg/5 mL, what is the volume of dopamine that we need?

So another formula that we need is:

$$\textbf{Amount of drug (mL)} = \frac{\textbf{Dose that you want (mg)} \times \textbf{Volume it is in (mL)}}{\textbf{Dose that it is in (mg)}}$$

So in our example

$$\textbf{Amount of drug (mL)} = \frac{\textbf{81 mg} \times \textbf{5 mL}}{\textbf{200 mg}}$$

Amount of drug (mL) = 2.025 mL

So we need 2.02 mL of dopamine to be made up to 50 mL in order to get our required concentration.

Cautionary note about dosing units of medication, that some are dosed in microgram/kg/min, as opposed to microgram/kg/hr. This is to do with the final units being too big!!!

Over the next few days Bobby remains stable with his blood pressure gradually increasing to a mean of 36. As a result the doctors wish to wean the dose of dopamine so as to stop it. They wish to wean it in increments of 1 microgram/kg/min every 4 hours depending on how well Bobby maintains his blood pressure.

By what rate would each decrease of 1 microgram/kg/min equate to?

Bobby is commenced on oral feeds and is weaned off his morphine and the ventilator. He is reloaded on caffeine citrate at 20 mg/kg. His CRP has reduced but his blood had grown Group B *Streptococci* which was shown to be sensitive to benzylpenicillin and gentamicin. He has to complete a 7-day course of antibiotics.

The numbers related to ventilation

A brief discussion follows which clearly needs to be expanded on via PDP activity should more number-related knowledge be required. Mechanical ventilation allows the work of breathing to be taken on by a machine known as ventilator. There are many types of ventilator which do more or less work for the baby depending upon their clinical condition, age, gestation, blood gas result or oxygen requirement to name but a few. Ventilators will have readings which the nurse documents as part of her hourly (or more frequent) observations, these observations can be used to gain a clinical 'picture' of how well or not a baby is doing and whether support needs to be increased or can be reduced ("weaned"). Data such as peak inspiratory pressure (PiP), positive end expiratory pressure (PEEP), fraction of inspired oxygen (FiO_2), inspiratory time, expiratory time, mean airway pressure (MAP), tidal volume and rate. To calculate the minute volume you take the tidal volume × rate and divide by 1000 to get L/min (the answer will be expressed as a decimal). So the normal tidal volume of a neonate is 4–7 L/min. For Bobby, if he was on a rate of 40 breaths per minute (bpm) on the ventilator, would be expected to have a minute volume (MV) of 0.21–0.37 L/min.

That is, 4–7 mL × 1.35 Kg × 40 bpm then divide by 1000 to give L/min.

Outcomes in relation to Bobby

Following on from the intensive care Bobby needed in the early days of his young life he progressed well with his feeds and was fully fed on EBM of 150 mL/kg by 10 days of age.

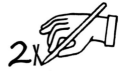

How much does this work out to be at a weight of 1.35 kg, hourly?

Bobby continued to put on weight and reached his birthweight at day 14, and he was commenced on multivitamin drops of 0.6 mL/day. He is now able to tolerate feeds every 2 hours – what volume of feed does he require?

Note that generally speaking the birthweight is always used to calculate feeds and medications until it is exceeded.

When Bobby is 5 weeks old in nursery the same principles for calculating fluids (by now this is full enteral feeds) apply. Weighing 1.87 kg and requiring 165 mL/kg/day, Bobby's fluid requirements = 308.5 mL of total feed volume. He is now being fed three hourly so the total is divided by 8 = 38.56 mL which in the case of feeds can be rounded up to 39 mL. IV fluids would not be rounded up by this much as infusion pumps are able to deliver fluid within two decimal places. Also, for tiny babies rounding up by let us say 0.5 mL every hour would equal an extra 12 mL per day – in the case of the 500 g 23-week gestation baby who may only require 60 mL/kg = 30 mL/day so that extra 12 mL is nearly half as much again. Fluid overload could result or further electrolyte imbalance.

CONCLUDING COMMENTS

This chapter has focused in on the numbers related to the care of a neonate which cover all the basic skills covered in earlier chapters and should give you the confidence to manage the complex fluid and medicines management needed for children like Bobby where numerical accuracy is vital for safe and effective practice. The next chapter will consider how children of different ages and abilities develop number sense and how nurses can work with children where knowledge of numbers is integral to their self-care using the example of a child with type 1 diabetes mellitus.

Chapter 7

CHILD DEVELOPMENT AND NUMBER SENSE

Numeracy in Children's Nursing, First Edition. Arija Parker
© 2015 John Wiley & Sons, Ltd. Published 2015 by John Wiley & Sons Ltd.

LEARNING FOCUS

To explore the world of numeracy skills development in children and young people.

LEARNING OUTCOMES

By the end of this chapter you should be able to:

- Define number sense
- Build on existing child development knowledge and develop some insight into how children learn about numbers
- Reflect on how this impacts on professional nursing practice
- Revise and update your knowledge of children and young people's diabetes care and management
- Identify and define your personal learning trajectory in relation to basic numeracy skills learning and teaching – where you plan to go from here

CASE SCENARIO 9

Peter Pascal (12), who is known by a nickname Pi by his family, was diagnosed with Type 1 diabetes mellitus when he was 2. He is under the care of a paediatrician with a specialist interest in diabetes and a children's diabetes specialist nurse who are based at Arch Mede Hospital. He lives on the outskirts of Pythagoras and is in the first year of High School. His symptoms at diagnosis were polydipsia and polyuria which were noticed by his mum, though he had also lost a lot of weight. His blood sugar at diagnosis was 19 mmols/L. He has only had one admission to hospital since he was diagnosed, when he was 9, following an acute illness that led to an episode of diabetic ketoacidosis (DKA), which resulted in a hospital stay of 4 days. He lives with his mum and stepdad and twin sister, Poppy, who is fit and well though worried about 'getting' diabetes. The following chapter will focus in on the specific aspects of Pi's life with diabetes as well as consider his needs at different developmental stages also considering his needs as he moves from childhood into adolescence.

Numerical data will be included though not in the same format as with other chapters because this chapter has a very different content and is mostly based on literacy skills to illustrate problems rather than discuss specific numeracy skills as in the previous chapters. Needless to say though, numerical problems will still be encountered along the way. The focus is also very much on community settings and the nursing roles of caring and teaching children and young people in home environments and school, which demonstrates a slight departure from what has been the norm so far.

TREE OF MATHS KNOWLEDGE

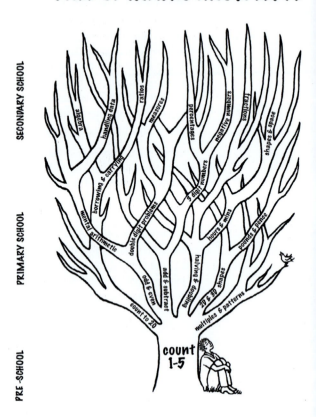

SECONDARY SCHOOL

PRIMARY SCHOOL

PRE-SCHOOL

algebra
handling data
ratios
measures
percentages
negative numbers
fractions
shapes & space
borrowing & carrying
3 digit numbers
mental arithmetic
double digit problems
hours & mins
pounds & pence
odd & even
add & subtract
halving & doubling
2D & 3D shapes
count to 20
multiples & patterns

count
1-5

INTRODUCTION

The focus of this chapter is to identify and explore how children comprehend and use numbers using a developmental approach using Pi's experiences from age 2 till 12 to explore how this impacts on his diabetes self-management. Reference has already been made in earlier chapters to how children understand and use number. This chapter will expand on and develop this information so as to aid our understanding of how to discuss numerical information with children. This will also aid us when teaching children the skills needed to manage their health effectively, thus reducing hospital admissions and promoting optimal health.

The UK education system and the use of Key Stages, will be used to assemble a framework of developmental stages in terms of numeracy development which should also give the nurse caring for children and young people some insight into what the abilities of each age group should be in relation to numerical ability. As with milestones and development stages these divisions are not discrete and children will vary in their development for all sorts of reasons. The chapter will start with a discussion about diabetes and its management, which will then be followed by an exploration of the child's world of numbers and numeracy skill acquisition, concluding with some suggestions on how this knowledge is useful for children's nursing practice. This chapter also serves as the concluding chapter of this book and so will give you the opportunity to examine where you have reached in your numeracy learning journey. Have you tamed the number beast and where do you plan to journey onwards to?

What is diabetes?

Defining diabetes

Diabetes mellitus is a condition in which the glucose level in the blood is higher than it should be, because the insulin-producing cells of the pancreas are destroyed by autoimmunity. Insulin is essential for processing glucose in the bloodstream and in its absence the blood glucose level increases and is excreted in urine (Hanas, 2012). The word 'diabetes' comes from the Greek word for 'siphon' or 'flowing through'. The word 'mellitus' comes from the Latin word for 'honeyed'. Diabetes mellitus has been known for thousands of years, having been described by the Ancient Egyptians and the Romans. There are two types which are distinguished by the need for insulin, – insulin-dependent diabetes mellitus (type 1) and non–insulin-dependent diabetes mellitus (type 2). Type 2 is also known as adult onset usually occurring after the age of 35 though increasingly it is becoming a disease of childhood due to increasing incidence of childhood obesity. The reason why this happens is due to insulin resistance and is usually treated with oral medication that aims to increase the body's sensitivity to insulin (Hanas, 2012).

Diabetes insipidus is a different condition that will not be discussed in this chapter. It is a very rare condition caused by the lack of a hormone needed to concentrate urine. This hormone is produced in the brain. Diabetes insipidus shares the name diabetes as it also results in the production of large quantities of urine, but has nothing to do with how the body manages glucose.

Key principles of type 1 diabetes management with a focus on numeracy skills

The key aspects of diabetes management include administering insulin, managing diet and monitoring condition (blood glucose levels, urine testing and HbA1c) within the context of a holistic healthy approach to lifestyle. Most aspects of care have a numeracy component to them as follows:

1. **Administering insulin**

    At diagnosis – Children, such as Pi at the age of 2, are given one, two or three insulin injections per day: these are usually injections of short-acting insulin or rapid-acting insulin analogue mixed with intermediate-acting insulin. The insulin preparations may be mixed by the child/parent/carer at the time of injection, as was the case for Pi 10 years ago when diabetes management was different with respect to insulin administration regimes.

    At school age – Children are usually commenced on a multiple daily injection regimen: the child has injections of short-acting insulin or rapid-acting insulin analogue before meals, together with one or more separate daily injections of intermediate-acting insulin or long-acting insulin analogue.

    As Pi moves into adolescence he is thinking about going onto an insulin pump – a continuous subcutaneous insulin infusion (insulin pump therapy): a programmable pump and insulin storage reservoir that gives a regular or continuous amount of insulin (usually in the form of a rapid-acting insulin analogue or short-acting insulin) by a subcutaneous needle or cannula (NICE, 2004).

Children and young people with type 1 diabetes using insulin injection regimens should be offered needles that are of an appropriate length for their body fat (short needles are appropriate for children and young people with less body fat (5 mm); longer needles are appropriate for children and young people with more body fat (8 mm or 12 mm)).

2. **Blood glucose monitoring and normal ranges (capillary)**
   Blood glucose levels are monitored using a blood glucose meter using a capillary sample of blood (gained by using a lancing device). Pi monitors his blood glucose before meals and whenever he has concerns about his blood sugar being high or too low. A preprandial (pre-meal) blood glucose should be between 4–5.9 mmol/L and postprandial (after meals) under 7.8 mmol/L. It is usually measured in mmol/L though can also be measured in mg/dL in the non-diabetic population.

3. **HbA1c monitoring and normal ranges**
   HbA1c is a measure of average blood glucose over a longer period of time and measures the amount of glucose that is bound to haemoglobin over the life span of a red blood cell (120 days). It has till recently been measured as a percentage and so measures the average blood glucose level over 3 months. Children and young people with type 1 diabetes and their families should be informed that the target for long-term glycaemic control is an HbA1c level of less than 7.5% without frequent disabling hypoglycaemia and that their care package should be designed to attempt to achieve this (NICE, 2004). Confusion can arise with units of measurement whereby at present it is measured in percentages though there will be different reference values in different laboratories (Hanas, 2010). The percentage way of reporting HbA1c values

is known as the Diabetes Control and Complications Trial (DCCT) unit, though there is now a move to use a new system of mmols/mol values are known as the International Federation of Clinical Chemistry (IFCC) units. It is recommended that people with diabetes try to keep their HbA1c levels below 48 mmols/mol (under the new units). Pi and his family do understand the value of the measure though are confused by the change in measure which is similar to the measure of blood glucose in mmol/L though obviously is not the same, that is, because of the volume in litres.

4. **Urine testing**

   This is no longer the primary testing required to monitor diabetic control. It is useful as a 'screening method' to determine when glucose is excreted and is also a useful test, though less accurate than a blood glucose, when it is impractical to do a blood glucose test (particularly for young children). It used to be the best way to measure for ketones (and high blood glucose), though blood strips for ketones are now available. When urine glucose is measured it reflects the average blood glucose level since the child last passed urine. It is measured as a percentage (Hanas, 2012).

5. **Monitoring carbohydrate intake**

   Monitoring carbohydrate and particularly carbohydrate counting is a way of matching insulin requirements with the amounts of carbohydrate that are eaten or drunk and leads to better diabetes control with greater flexibility and freedom of lifestyle (Diabetes UK). Whilst it takes time to master the skill it is argued that it is worth it in the long run. When Pi was diagnosed the emphasis was on healthy eating approaches though now as he is approaching adulthood and wants to be more in control and independent he is learning about carbohydrate counting.

Children and young people with type 1 diabetes and their families should be informed that they have the same basic nutritional requirements as other children and young people. The food choices of children and young people should provide sufficient energy and nutrients for optimal growth and development, with total daily energy intake being distributed as follows:

- carbohydrates – more than 50%
- protein – 10–15%
- fat – 30–35%.

The consumption of five portions of fruits and vegetables per day is also recommended. Neonates, infants and preschool children require individualised dietary assessment of their energy needs.

- **Glycaemic index**

Not only is advice offered about CHO intake but also glycaemic index (GI) needs to be taken into account.

Some foods and their glycaemic index.

Low GI	Medium GI	High GI
Apples, oranges, pears, peaches	Honey	Pure sugar (glucose)
Beans and lentils	Jam	White and wholemeal bread
Pasta (made from durum wheat)	Ice cream	Brown and white rice (cooked)
Porridge	Couscous	Cornflakes
Custard	New potatoes, peeled and boiled	Baked and mashed potato

Source: Diabetes UK

What is also worth mentioning is the impact of fibre – a higher percentage of fibre will cause the glucose to be absorbed more slowly. When carbohydrate counting, the amount of fibre should be subtracted from total carbohydrates if it is 5 g or more per 100 g. The GI and fibre content of food will not affect insulin requirements though will influence how insulin should be taken, that is, basal bolus, twice daily or via pump (Hanas, 2010).

6. Exercise

Children and young people with type 1 diabetes should be encouraged to monitor their blood glucose levels before and after exercise so that they can:

- Identify when changes in insulin or food intake are necessary
- Learn the glycaemic response to different exercise conditions
- Be aware of exercise-induced hypoglycaemia
- Be aware that hypoglycaemia may occur several hours after prolonged exercise.

Children and young people with type 1 diabetes, their parents and other carers should be informed that additional carbohydrate should be consumed as appropriate to avoid hypoglycaemia and that carbohydrate-based foods should be readily available during and after exercise.

This basic introduction to diabetes management, which does not cover all the aspects and detail of day-to-day care, identifies how important it is for children, young people and their families to understand the numbers that relate to management of their day-to-day health and well-being. To be able to do this they need to have the care explained to them by knowledgeable healthcare staff. The next section will explore how children learn about and use numbers in their lives.

Child development and number sense

This section will examine the development of number sense in children from preschool stage through to early adolescent stages. In light of this it is worth briefly exploring child development in general with a particular focus on learning and Aldgate et al's (2006) ecological model seems to be the most logical and succinct way of doing this.

What do we mean by growth and development?

Smith (2003) defines development as:

> '...the process by which an organism grows and changes through it's life span'.

So how can knowledge and understanding of child growth and development help assess a child's ability to do numeracy-related activities to help them both understand what is going on with their bodies as well as understand what the numbers mean? It will help you in: effective communication, advising and supporting parents, understanding of child behaviours, creating an environment to support the child's health and well-being, tailoring health promotion and making professional judgements.

Milestones *en route* to healthy growth and development

Aldgate et al. (2006) ecological model identify 'Milestones' as a term that recognises that:

- As children grow, and assuming they have been given appropriate parenting and support from others, their competencies and, consequently, confidence in different areas of development will change.
- For all children, development will be sequential – all children will gain competence in certain developmental tasks, in the same order but not necessarily at the same rate or age.

Child growth and development has been studied from many different perspectives such as: physical, cognitive, emotional, environmental, cultural and psychosocial. These are rather false separations as all of these are intertwined, however it can help to narrow the subject area to facilitate research and theory development. Some of the criticisms of child growth and development theories are their bias towards Western societal and cultural norms. Societal and cultural goals are very different across the globe and the same aspects apply to number skills acquisition, that is, the Chinese perspective and use of language where language used in relation to numbers ensures clearer understanding of what the numbers mean as discussed in Chapter 1. When thinking about the teaching of mathematics the changing environment and impact of technology has made a significant difference to how children learn, that is, use of computers, video games and internet compared with even 20 years ago which has an impact on us adults, both as parents and nurses when teaching children about numbers.

In terms of defining a starting point it is worth mentioning the work of Piaget as one of the main developmental theorists accessed in nurse education. Piaget's theories, as with most developmental theories, are divided into stages or phases. These are based on qualitative changes in behaviour over time and age and describe an invariant sequence of development. The rate of growth may differ but the order is always the same, where each stage has a structural cohesiveness – behaviour is consistent and coherent and stages form a hierarchy because each stage builds on earlier stages (Leather et al., cited in Wyse (2000)). Later discussion will highlight this 'building bricks' approach whereby it is vital for children to learn numericals in stages building on this prior learning as they progress through Key Stages.

The reason for mentioning the child development theories such as Piaget's is that they offer a basis for reasoning and evaluating how children learn, grow and develop and throw up many questions that form the basis for designing curricula that support learning and teaching. Are children under the age of 5 able to conceptualise what is a number? We clearly need to have some concept of the intellectual milestones so as to approximate dates to cognitive achievements. The theories offer us some guidance into how children think and learn and certainly gives us good information in relation to numerical ability seeing that all the tasks children participated in from the Piagetian perspective and in Piaget's experiments were mathematical in nature (and will be mentioned later in this discussion). With respect to number in the animal kingdom Sousa (2007) argues that animals can recognise a certain number of objects. The arguments then is that why cannot infants do the same so negating arguments that have been made that children have to wait till they are 4/5 to gain the abilities that animals possess. Do children have an innate number sense from birth?

Child Development in relation to acquisition of numerical skills

Whilst there is a great body of evidence to suggest that we should not divide childhood up into distinct stages this is the approach that we use in health and social care and particularly in relation to education so we will look at the UK approach to education and curricular development, that is, preschool nursery or kindergarten, primary school (age 4–11) which is usually divided into primary and junior stages and then secondary school from 11–16 from where students will usually go on for further education in colleges or A level study in other centres. These are reflected in the key stage approach used in the national curriculum going from the preschool strategy through Key Stages 1–4 up to GCSE level (examinations taken at age 15–16).

Whilst, as already discussed at length in this book, there is a close relationship between literacy and numeracy the curriculum will be examined in relation to a child's development from the numbers perspective primarily.

Preschool development

The key characteristics of a preschoolers development are:

- Attachment to caregivers
- Gross and fine motor skills
- Communication and early language
- Increasingly complex expressions of emotion
- Differentiation of self from others
- Self-control and compliance

Source: Aldgate et al. (2006) ecological model

The issue around whether formal mathematics should be taught to preschoolers is a contestable fact where gut reactions would say that they are too young, though Sousa

(2007) argues that we should take opportunities to work with innate number sense and start developing these skills at this stage. He argues that mathematics activities should raise children's intuitive number sense and pattern recognition abilities to an explicit level of awareness. Number sense has been mentioned frequently so what follow are some definitions.

A person's ability to recognise that something has changed in a small collection when without that person's knowledge an object has been added or removed from the collection (Danzig, 1967).

Numbers have meanings as any other lived experience such as language or music. We are born with an innate number sense. This skill is possessed by many animals and contributes to our ability to survive and communicate with each other (Sousa, 2007).

As already mentioned earlier, Piaget (1953) argued that children do not develop a conceptual understanding of arithmetic till they are 7 or 8 years old. Stage 1 of his theory (sensorimotor covering 0–2 years) identifies that infants are born with innate reflexes such as sucking and grasping. These innate schemata (where a schema is the discovery and description of mental structures), progressively develop in response to new experiences into new schemata via the process of accommodation. When a schema matches experiences new information is assimilated. The child is totally egocentric and learning to distinguish self from the rest of the world and explore objects and toys by sucking and handling, so by 8 months of age they are developing their sensory and motor skills. By the end of the 18-month period a child will be starting to think symbolically, that is, with the use of early language.

There is not much difference between what Piaget observed and theorised as compared with other theorists, though other writers do argue that human infants are born with an innate number sense. This is contradicted by writers such as Sousa (2007). He argues that the ability to count and the ability to use and manipulate symbols that represent numerical quantities is part of innate number sense.

Subitising, where you recognise the number in a small collection immediately without counting and applies to four or fewer objects is something that young children can do. Once you go beyond four you have to start counting or estimating. There are two types: perceptual, where it is purely recognition of a number, whilst the conceptual aspect allows you to know the number by recognising familiar patterns, that is, dots on dice or by using fingers to count out (Clements, 1999).

Wynn (1990, cited in Sousa, 2007) found that by 30 months, children can understand through observation what the process of counting is. By age 3 most children recognise that there are separate words to describe quantities of something. It is complex - -they have to get the correct sequence to the point where they recognise that the last word in the sequence is the total number of objects. This is called the CARDINAL PRINCIPLE.

Going back to Piaget's theory at Stage 2 (pre-operational ages 2–7 years) toddlers can distinguish between self and objects. They still cannot conceive the idea of experiencing others viewpoint and are unable to consider two aspects of the same situation at the same time.

To see the list of video clips of some of Piaget's experiments and the milestones achieved in the early stages of childhood.

Even though children see the change process, that is, pouring a drink from short, fat glass to tall, thin glass they do not believe that the same amount is in the glass as before. They learn by using repetition, that is, can listen to the same story time and time again or doing the same jigsaw for the millionth time. They do not understand reversibility in relation to mathematical problems, that is, $2 + 3 = 5$ is the same as $5 - 3 = 2$. They cannot reason beyond the observable and lack the ability to make deductions or generalisations and their thought is dominated by what they see, hear or otherwise experience. At the end of the period they are only able to begin to deal with issues of weight, length, size and time, that is, understanding what is today and what is tomorrow? Piaget argues that the idea that changing the items in a collection does not change the number does not happen until the age of 5.

Does this mean that we should not start numeracy education at preschool settings or at home? Van Nes and van Erde (2010) argue that not only do young children (4–6) have number sense they also have spatial sense, which relates to the ability to grasp the external world – spatial visualisation, special orientation and shape (Clements and Saraman cited in van Nes and van Erde (2010)). Their work and research emphasises that we should make best use with respect to early years, teaching in developing these spatial skills. The teaching role is all around using a Vygotskian approach where you coach and guide using a bottom-up approach starting with the individual child working one-to-one with an adult.

4-year-olds are able to subitise and do finger counting and start looking at and defining quantities, that is, two stacks of bricks identifying which is more or less (and this applies to time and use of money) They will know each word for a number occurs in a fixed sequence and each only applies to one object in a collection. They also know that the last number word is the total number of objects in that collection. They can count to five and some can count to ten (Sousa, 2007).

The Department for Education (2014) statutory framework for Early Years Foundation Stage education from birth to 5, identified that children should be offered opportunities to improve their skills in counting, understanding and using numbers, calculating simple addition and subtraction problems and to describe shapes, spaces and measures. Is this a reasonable expectation?

Specifically children should be given opportunities to learn to:

- Count reliably from 1 to 20, place them in order and identify which number is one more or one less than a given number.
- Add and subtract two single digit numbers and count on or back to find an answer.

- Solve problems including doubling, halving and sharing.
- Using everyday language talk about size, weight, capacity, position, distance, time and money to compare quantities and objects and to solve problems.
- Recognise, create and describe patterns.

This reflects the approach taken by the NCTM (2006) though their focus is more on the shapes, pattern recognition and developing spatial relationships rather than being able to do addition and subtraction, which from the evidence appears to be more suitable for a primary school setting. They suggest that children should explore number by counting objects and using counting on methods to explore the principles of addition, that is, by counting spaces and moving on in board games. They should be looking at shapes to explore properties, develop measurement skills, recognise patterns and analyse data, that is, sorting objects by colour, size and shape through interesting activities like watching bean plants sprout and grow.

From a nursing perspective this does give us some idea with regard to what 3–5-year olds are able to comprehend when we introduce numbers into our discussions either via play or when discussing health-related issues, that is, how much and what to eat, how to use a pain assessment tool or why we are pricking their finger to measure blood glucose and counting the number of clicks to administer insulin as some examples.

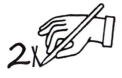

Pi was 2 when he was diagnosed and at a stage of development where he was very active, very uncooperative and very fussy in his eating pattern whereas on some days he would sit and eat with his sister and family though on other days would refuse to eat. What advice could you offer mum in relation to managing blood sugars and diet?

At diagnosis Pi's mum, who was a single parent at the time, really struggled both to deal with the psychological aspects and impact of diabetes on family life. She was also caring for Pi's twin sister, Poppy, who was really confused by what was going on, especially as she had to stay with her auntie for a week whilst Pi and mum were in hospital at diagnosis.

Taking diabetes management back 10 years, whilst in hospital for a full week, mum was taught to mix insulin – a short- and long-acting insulin in an insulin syringe with short needle – administer it, carbohydrate counting, blood glucose monitoring, urine testing etc. She needed lots of support and advice from the dietician to manage what can often be perceived as difficult toddler behaviour, such as trying half a glass of juice or milk at breakfast time so that when the blood glucose level has risen a bit his appetite will have improved, which works well and Pi still does at the age of 12, when he does not feel like eating breakfast before school. She was advised to never force-feed Pi and try to play down the emphasis on food, though this is very difficult for parents of toddlers whether they have diabetes or not. Mum did not have a rigid meal regime in place at home so decided to take a grazing approach, that is, lots of small regular meals throughout the day in the same way that she did prior to diagnosis to keep a routine that worked well before (even though he did not always eat) (Hanas, 2010).

Mum did become very obsessed with reading food labels, where it was a struggle to understand the information, seeing as food labelling was not as good 10 years ago, and found the food tables produced by diabetes charities are really helpful in terms of determining amounts and portion sizes for Pi. At diagnosis she did find the volume of information she had to take on overwhelming as well as new skills she had to develop. She was also really worried by the numbers and getting insulin amounts wrong when drawing up and measuring using insulin syringes.

Specifics of diabetes care at the age of 2:

Insulin amounts – 0.5×11.3 kg $= 5.65$ units per day

It was administered as 4 units before breakfast and 1.5 units pre-evening meal.

This is administered in a premix insulin formula (biphasic insulin aspart) – using fast-acting insulin and a longer acting one in proportion of 30% insulin aspart and 70% insulin aspart protamine these days, though at time of diagnosis he was using an insulin syringe with mum having to mix insulins from two separate vials.

Human insulin analogue – insulin aspart and insulin lispro have a fast onset (10–20 minutes) and short action duration (2–5 hours). This is particularly useful for young children where fast onset is needed and intake of food is unpredictable or may be refused (BNF for children, 2012). It can be given before or immediately after food which then makes it easier to adjust dosages and prevent hypoglycaemia (low blood glucose) when children's eating patterns are unpredictable.

The protamine part contains isophane insulin which is longer acting and the onset of action is at 1–2 hours and maximal effect at 4–12 hours with a duration of 16–35 hours.

In Pi's case, at newly diagnosed stage he was on a twice daily regime.

The following table shows a sample of his blood glucose readings in the early stages of diagnosis.

Blood glucose levels at diagnosis (measured in mmol/L).

Day	Before breakfast	Before midday meal	Before evening meal	Before supper	Key events/notes
Monday	5.2	4.8	10.0	19.0	Honeymoon period
Tuesday	6.3	7.3	3.2	7.2	Hypo when out playing in the garden
Wednesday	7.2	4.2	7.3	7.8	
Thursday	3.9	9.2	4.6	4.3	
Friday	9.8	7.7	5.3	6.9	

Advice given to parent

Mum was advised to check urine for ketones if blood glucose was >15mmol/L. If 2+ or more, contact the diabetes specialist nurses. If below 4 mmol/L, Pi to have 100 mL of sugary drink, wait 10 minutes and recheck blood sugar to ensure that it is 4 mmol/L and then have a carbohydrate snack. This serves to illustrate the complexity of managing the diabetes care of a child as well as being mum to an active toddler. Numeracy skills for the adult are paramount, that is, using dipsticks, using sticks and glucose meter, telling the time measuring out drinks etc. How often do we actually assess the numeracy knowledge of adults as patients and parents?

Define the term: Honeymoon period

Children and young people with newly diagnosed type 1 diabetes should be informed that they may experience a partial remission phase (or 'honeymoon period') during which a low dosage of insulin (0.5 units/kg body weight/day) may be sufficient to maintain an HbA1c level of less than 7% (NICE, 2004).

Children and young people with newly diagnosed type 1 diabetes should be offered a structured programme of education covering the aims of insulin therapy, delivery of insulin, self-monitoring of blood glucose, the effects of diet, physical activity and intercurrent illness on glycaemic control, and the detection and management of hypoglycaemia (NICE, 2004).

Middle childhood development

The key characteristics of middle childhood development are:

- Developing friendships with peers.
- Increasing complex physical capabilities and coordination.
- Capable of long periods of concentration.
- Moods becoming more stable, beginning of capacity for empathy and worry.
- Developing sense of values (right versus wrong, what is fair, etc.).

- Beginning to regulate behaviour appropriately in different settings.
- Able to communicate ideas and expression of wishes.
- Literacy and numeracy skills become established.

Source: Aldgate et al. (2006) ecological model

Primary Key Stage 1

The National Strategy, Primary Framework (DfES, 2006) identifies five key theme strands:

1. Problem-solving
2. Representing
3. Enquiring
4. Reasoning
5. Communicating

The framework encourages the importance for children in using key skills, that is, seeking patterns, making connections and recognising relationships. Are they able to do this? The emphasis is on number, shape, space and measures for Key Stage 1.

From Piaget's theory at stage 3 (concrete operational 7–11) children are now using more integrated and stable patterns of thought. What he defines as 'operations' are the key, that is, they can decentre and can conserve, so are able to consider a wide variety of problems, though function best when have concrete knowledge of the problem under consideration. Thinking becomes logical and children can perform the mental operation of reversibility and can attend to several aspects of a situation at once and overcome egocentrism. Children can classify, sort, order and organise facts about the world and use it in problem-solving. Volume, weight and number remain the same though outward appearance has changed. They can solve problems in a concrete, systematic fashion based on their perception. Reasoning is inductive in that they cannot work from the abstract. His work has led the way in education to argue that children do not develop a conceptual understanding of maths till they are 7 or 8 (Sousa, 2007). The UK system clearly starts the process of acquiring numeracy skills at a much younger age.

Some of the skills to be acquired:

- Problem-solving using numbers, communicate using the correct language symbols associated with number, present results in an organised way
- Count up to 20 gradually extending to 100 and beyond
- Create and describe number patterns learning to do addition and subtraction and the patterns of multiples of 2, 5 and 20, odd and even numbers to 30 and then beyond
- Halving and doubling
- In relation to mental maths – learn number facts and carry out simple calculations
- Be able to describe the properties of common 2D and 3D shapes, recognise right angles, estimate size of objects by using comparisons.

They will be learning addition, subtraction, multiplication, division, fractions, decimals, percentages, ratio and proportions as they proceed from the reception through (at the age of 4 or 5) to year 6 following the UK model of primary education. Will all children be able to acquire all these numeracy skills?

To introduce some new numeracy-related terms to the discussion, 'representing' means the way in which we can represent real life or concrete situations in mathematical language, pictures or symbols. It is the basis of the process called mathematical modelling. Sousa (2007) argues that children are able to understand the commutative rule, that is, that $a + b = b + a$ at around the age of 5. He argues that a significant change in thinking occurs at around the age of 5 where children start developing skills learned in earlier years into a hierarchy.

Six-year-old children have developed a mental number line where they have developed a central cognitive conceptual and structure for whole numbers and they can use counting skills in a broad range of new contexts. They can read hours on clock, know which two identically sized monetary values is worth the most, as two examples (Sousa, 2007).

Sousa (2007) discussing estimation argues that this is an important skill to have and is an extension to the brain's natural ability to subitise. Children are very quick to notice if halves of a cake are not equal when asked to share though within maths teaching the emphasis on getting the answer right seems to account for poor estimation skills that persist into adulthood. As nurses, we are so focused on getting the correct answer we are unwilling to estimate to check that our answer is correct. It is all about finding a balance between allowing children to find their own ways of completing numeracy tasks so developing an understanding of how, what and why as opposed to rote learning using one method. Most children find addition easy to understand though multiplication is much more complex and these problems can persist into adulthood. You need to understand four related concepts – quantity, problem situations requiring multiplication, equal group and units relevant to multiplication.

Whilst at primary school children move into junior level and Key Stage 2.

The emphasis within the National Curriculum is on number, space, shape and measures and handling data (DfEE, 2004) and children should be able to do the following:

- Make connections in mathematics
- Break down complex problems into simpler steps, and select appropriate equipment (including use of ICT)
- Count on and back in tens or hundreds from any two or other digit number
- Recognise and continue number sequences including the use of negative numbers
- Recognise and describe number patterns including multiples of 2, 5 and 10
- Recognise prime number to 20 and square number up to 10×10

- Understand unit fractions, simple equivalent fractions and simplify by cancelling
- Recognise equivalence between decimal and fraction forms, find percentages, solve simple problems involving ratio and direct proportion
- Understand and use decimal notation for tenths and hundredths
- Round numbers to one or two decimal places
- Work with 4-number operations and use of inverses, find remainders after division and understand the use of brackets to determine the order of operations
- Know all the addition and subtraction facts for each number to 20
- Multiplication facts to 10×10 and be able use them quickly
- Multiply and divide.

In addition to advancing skills in relation to shape and measurement and handling data, 8-year-old children are able to manipulate two number lines so are able to work with two variables – they can understand place value and can use mental arithmetic to solve double digit addition problems. They can read hours and minutes on the clock and can solve monetary problems where you might be dealing with pounds and pence. 10-year-old children can manage two number lines structure and include a third variable and are developing a deeper understanding of the whole number system and can compute three- digit numbers and understand the principles of borrowing and carrying. They are able to work out which time is longer when working in hours and minutes.

What is Pi up to during middle childhood?

He is doing well at school and managing his diabetes whilst at school though mum takes over when he gets home. He is having a packed lunch so that his mum can continue carbohydrate counting and manage his diabetes from home whilst giving him some independence with respect to monitoring his blood glucose and administering his own insulin.

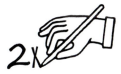

Pi at the age of 9 weighs 35 kg and so what are his insulin requirements now?

His insulin regimen has changed to basal bolus insulin therapy using a pen device – short-acting insulin three times a day and long-acting insulin before bed given in a 3, 3, 3, 8 regime. The long-acting one is the background insulin that works day and night to ensure that it is the basal part of the therapy. The bolus part is the short-acting insulin which is normally given before food at breakfast, lunch and tea/dinner. This allows for much greater flexibility. At the age of 9 Pi is learning about experimenting with the help of diabetes nurse with respect to changes in amounts of food that he is eating particularly in relation to the amount of exercise he does. He is a keen sportsman and plays for his town's under-10's football team. So, as an example, his blood glucose was 5.2 mmol/L the evening before so he was running low. He attended a football tournament all day on Sunday and then had a difficult week where ordinarily his blood sugars are on a fairly even keel with respect to the aim of running between 4–8 mmol/L. He rarely has hypoglycaemic episodes and usually only goes as high as 11 mmol usually before lunchtime.

Pi and Poppy's favourite numeracy joke

Pi: Why are you scratching your head?

Delta: I have those numeracy bugs again

Pi: Numeracy bugs – what are they?

Delta: Well some people call them head lice

Pi: Then why do you call them numeracy bugs?

Delta: Because they add to my misery, subtract from my pleasure, divide my attention and multiply like crazy!

Pi's blood glucose levels the week before admission to hospital.

Day	Before breakfast	Before lunch	Before evening meal	Before bed	Key events/ notes
Monday	3.5	11.4	3.6/5.4	3.2/ 19.1	Ate two bananas and some chocolates before bed as extras to counteract low blood sugars
Tuesday	7.8	14.4	17.1	4.4	Swimming lesson
Wednesday	5.8	14.2	17	4.4	
Thursday	6.3	10.6	8.3	5.9	
Friday	5.6	12.6	11	7.1	
Saturday	9.0	8.7	11.2	11.7	Not feeling well – did not go to football training
Sunday	11	12.6	14	17	Complaining of cough and runny nose

The table shows Pi's blood glucose levels the week before he was admitted to the ward with DKA. He was more active than usual in this week and started complaining of a sore throat at the beginning of the week which became full blown upper respiratory tract infection (URTI) by the end of the week. Mum was not sure what to do and just hoped for the best and Pi did not have the confidence to give extra insulin to counteract the effects of increased metabolic impact and lack of insulin. He prefers to be told what to do rather than try to work out what he should be doing so he can follow the rules his mum gives though does find it difficult to problem solve and would definitely not experiment by giving himself variable doses of insulin.

Diabetic ketoacidosis

Whilst the purpose of this book is not to focus in on conditions in detail it does allow us to explore some of the numerical data that makes it easier to understand why certain things happen from a pathophysiological perspective and what is happening when he presents in A&E and then on the ward with DKA.

The core information that relates to the management of DKA appears in Section 3 on the website.

Arterial blood gases

A normal pH is between 7.35 and 7.45 and indicates when the body is in acid–base balance. This is all based on the behaviour of hydrogen ions and during a period of ill health this fine balance can be tipped with a pH below 7.35 with hydrogen ions increasing (acidosis or acidaemia) or go above 7.45 with hydrogen concentration decreasing resulting in alkalosis or alkalaemia.

Normal ranges pH: 7.35–7.45

$PaCO_2$: 4.0–6.0

Sodium bicarbonate (HCO_3): 222–226

The units of measurement are in kilopascals which can be converted from mmHg by diving by 7.5.

The pH scale represented visually.

Concentration of hydrogen ions compared with distilled water	The pH scale	Examples of solutions and pH
1/10,000,000	14	Caustic soda
1/1,000,000	13	Bleach
1/100,000	12	Soapy water
1/10,000	11	Household ammonia (11.9)
1/1000	10	Milk of magnesia (10.5)
1/100	9	Toothpaste (9.9)
1/10	8	Baking soda (8.4), seawater, eggs
0	7	Pure water
10	6	Urine, milk
100	5	Acid rain, coffee
1000	4	Tomato juice
10,000	3	Orange juice, soft drinks
100,000	2	Lemon juice (2.3), vinegar (2.9)
1,000,000	1	Hydrochloric acid from stomach lining (1)
10,000,000	0	Battery acid

See the website links to DKA guidelines and the calculations required to manage insulin and fluid requirements.

On discharge from hospital Pi went back to his usual basal bolus insulin regime

Children and young people with type 1 diabetes using multiple daily insulin regimens should be informed that injection of rapid-acting insulin analogues before eating (rather than after eating) reduces postprandial blood glucose levels and thus helps to optimise blood glucose control (NICE, 2004).

Adolescent development

This will be dealt with briefly because as you can see most numerical skills are learned at Key Stages 1 and 2 and then consolidated and practised further to Key Stage 3 and beyond to GCSE and then to further and higher education. As already discussed in relation to adult education and working with numbers in Chapter 1 the issues around why many young people are unable to read, write and work with numbers is an issue that warrants discussion though this is beyond the scope of this book. This section also allows you to bridge the transition from the focus on basic numeracy skills to now start reflecting and planning on where you go from here in your numeracy learning.

The key characteristics of adolescent development are:

- Forming a cohesive sense of self-identity.
- Increasing ability to reason about hypothetical events.
- Forming close friendships within and across gender.
- Academic achievement (learning skills required for further education and work).
- Frequently questioning the belief system with which brought up.
- Period of experimentation.

Source: Aldgate et al. (2006) ecological model

Secondary Key Stage 3

The emphasis moves on from what has gone before and is on number, algebra, shape, space and measures and handling data (DfEE, 2004). In Piaget's stage 4 (formal operational at 11 years +) young people are developing abstract and logical thought, they can form and test hypotheses, theorise and criticise, have adaptability and flexibility and can think in an abstract way. They may confuse the ideal with the practical, though can deal with and resolve most contradictions in the world.

Pi as he moves into adolescence and on to adulthood

Pi (12) is in his first year at secondary school and now weighs 44 kg.

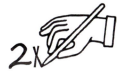

What are his insulin requirements?

At this stage of life it is worth taking a more holistic approach to self-management where numeracy and literacy skills are clearly linked and go hand in hand with the ability to problem solve and deal with many new problems linked to increased independence.

Skills needed to manage diabetes effectively:

1. Understanding of target blood glucose levels.
2. Ability to apply all aspects of basic carbohydrate counting.
3. Understanding of the action of insulin and the basal-bolus insulin concept.
4. Willingness and ability to keep adequate records.
5. Ability to identify patterns from records and adjust insulin requirements accordingly.
6. Understand how illness and exercise will impact on glycaemia control and manage accordingly.

To be able to acquire these skills he needs to have good literacy and numeracy skills, besides a willingness to comply to complex treatment and diabetes management regimes, as Pi becomes an adolescent and strives for independence and self-management of his diabetes. The team caring for him at Arch Mede Hospital are also working with the recommendations from the RCN and starting transitional arrangements as he moves towards adulthood (RCN, 2004).

Reflect on your own practice

Have you ever thought about the numeracy ability of the child, young person or parent whom you are educating or teaching? Does this change the approach you will take when putting a teaching programme together when teaching skills such as PEG feeding, home administration of intravenous medication or diabetes management? Write a short reflection to add to your professional portfolio.

CONCLUDING COMMENTS

This chapter has considered how children and young people learn about numbers and how this impacts on their self-management in relation to health and well-being. It also identifies the numeracy skills learned by linking them to the Key Stages via National Curriculum (2004). This should allow you to consider your role as a nurse teaching self-management skills to children and their families. This now leads us to the end of the book and the concluding comments, self-evaluation and plans for future numeracy-related practice that follow.

Chapter 8

WHERE DO I GO FROM HERE?

Concluding comments for this book
and your numeracy journey

Numeracy in Children's Nursing, First Edition. Arija Parker
© 2015 John Wiley & Sons, Ltd. Published 2015 by John Wiley & Sons Ltd.

LEARNING FOCUS

Moving onwards in children and young people's nursing practice with competence, in comfort and with confidence.

LEARNING OUTCOMES

By the end of this chapter you should be able to:

- Plan your future in relation to numeracy practice and education
- Identify further sources of information to allow for further practice
- Focus in on specialist areas of practice including specialist children's nursing practice, education, research and management

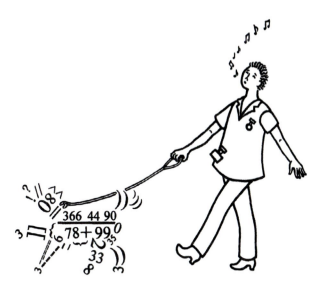

Have you tamed the 'number beast' and are you now walking this friendly numeracy dog?

The focus of this book has been on developing the basic numeracy skills that will enable nurses and other healthcare workers, who care for children and young people, to 'calculate competently, confidently and comfortably' and within the nursing context as defined as the motto of this book in Chapter 1.

At this stage it is to be hoped that all readers feel that they 'can do maths' or at the least feel more confident in their approach, so what follows are some suggestions to develop these skills further. It has no doubt been realised that practice is the key. If numeracy problems are not encountered frequently in clinical areas the key is to continue practising using the wealth of resources that are out there on the world wide web some of which can be accessed via the ONE website and resource.

The skills developed, that is, counting, use of and conversion of SI units, addition, subtraction, multiplication, division, use of fractions, percentages, ratios and proportion, use of formulae in relation to nursing practice in general as well as calculating medicine dosages offers you the basic skills that underpin more complex practice so there is great scope of exploring more complex scenarios relating to all the specialities in children's nursing practice (not just neonatal practice), as well as those related to research and management scenarios.

The ONE website contains some further practice examples as well as website links to allow you to explore the whole world of numeracy, not only from a nursing perspective. There will be a web resource out there to support your learning style and enable you to continue practising.

This book forms the base block of numeracy practice if you imagine a tower of building blocks, as identified in Chapter 7, when looking at how children learn numeracy skills – as they do so you have also used this approach. What you can now start doing is climbing up the tower and expanding your numeracy repertoire of skills which is particularly important if you want to progress in your nursing or healthcare career. Numbers will follow you on this journey and can become more complex or at least different as you change career direction.

The need to move further beyond this book is clear. With respect to the reading of research and evidence, numeracy knowledge can develop further because some statistical skills are vital. This is an essential requirement of all undergraduate programmes so all nursing students need to have a basic ability to read and interpret statistical information. One person who has not featured in this book and appears here at the end is someone who was more than a competent mathematician – that is, Florence Nightingale. It is not a stretch of the imagination to call Miss Nightingale a mathematician. She was using statistics as part of her work in designing hospital wards. She also introduced the process of triage into ways of working and organising care.

For those of you that are interested in nursing history and relationship to mathematics here are some web links to sources that explore Miss Nightingale's work in mathematics:

http://plus.maths.org/content/florence-nightingale-compassionate-statistician

http://malini-math.blogspot.co.uk/2009/11/florence-nightingales-contribution-to.html

Florence Nightingale the passionate statistician:
https://www.sciencenews.org/article/florence-nightingale-passionate-statistician

Great animation of some of her work and diagrams:
https://www.sciencenews.org/pictures/mathtrek/112608/nightingale.swf

As with the link to research all nurses will take on some management-related work so numeracy skills need to incorporate audit work, budgeting responsibilities, rostering and other basic accountancy skills so again adding greater confidence and use numbers in different contexts. Chapter 6 explored higher level numeracy skills as they apply to calculation and interpreting clinical data that apply to more specialist areas of children and young people's nursing practice. So more complex calculation will be encountered in more diverse, acute and high dependency care settings, that is, PICU, burns units and accident and emergency settings. In conclusion please return to the PDP templates and identify where you want your numeracy journey to take you next!

It is time to reflect on your progress to date and decide how to maintain and build on the numeracy skills learned and developed!

- Use the PDP template to identify your progress and plan further actions and activities that will allow you to practice, practice and practice!

The other important feature of this book is to consider the needs of children, young people and their families from a numbers perspective. Not only do we need to be able to calculate confidently – we also need to be able to teach these skills to children and adults alike. Chapter 7 has outlined some of the issues that need to be considered when thinking about children's numeracy ability and should enhance the teaching of skills to families who are increasingly caring for children with many more complex needs in community settings with support from nurses and other healthcare professionals. The book and website in particular identify some number-related play resources and books that can be used to distract and entertain children.

As a final concluding statement it is to be hoped that you can see where our numeracy skills base sits in our practice as children and young people's nurses where we need to celebrate numbers and be confident, comfortable and competent in our practice to provide care that is compassionate and caring.

Answers

CHAPTER 1 The Role of Numeracy in Nursing and Healthcare Practice

The missing prime numbers

2	3	5	7	11	13
17	19	23	29	31	37
41	43	47	53	59	61
67	71	73	79	83	89
97	101	103	107	109	113

Answer to why 1 does not count as a prime number: A prime number by definition is a number greater than one so one does not count. As defined above also the definition of a 'prime' number is one that has two factors: itself and 1. So the number 1, having only one factor, itself, does not meet the definition. The number 1 is not considered a prime number, although it is a unique integer.

CHAPTER 2 Counting and Measuring

Time

- 420 seconds
- 75 minutes
- 37 minutes
- 14.03 hours

Weight conversions

- 0.675 kg
- 1010 mg
- 7500 micrograms
- 0.015 mg

The abbreviated form of litre (L) should be used so it does not get confused with the number 1.

Predicting Banita's height at the age of 9 – by addition – 49 cm + 25 cm + 13 cm + 9 + 5 + 5 + 5 + 5 + 5 = 126 cm

Calculating Banita's weight using two formulas – 18 kg

Conversion of Banita's birth weight in pounds and ounces to kg – convert pounds and ounces into ounces = 102 and then convert 2.2 pounds into ounces = 34 and divide 102 by 34 to get the amount in kilograms = 3 kg

Estimated weight at the age of 5 using weight gain assessment (lower end of range) – 17.4 kg

Numeracy in Children's Nursing, First Edition. Arija Parker.
© 2015 John Wiley & Sons, Ltd. Published 2015 by John Wiley & Sons Ltd.

Calculating body surface area:
0.725 m² from BNF, 0.72 m² from formula (rounded to two decimal places)

Peak Expiratory Flow Rates

- 150
- 275
- 410

CHAPTER 3 Basic numeracy skills underpinning children and young people's nursing practice

Adding numbers: Add the following numbers together

- $59 + 82 = 141$
- $773 + 94 = 867$
- $71189 + 3901 = 75090$
- $7.5 + 9.1 = 16.6$
- $75.82 + 6.731 = 82.551$
- $700.821 + 3.21 = 704.031$

Subtracting numbers: Subtract the following numbers

- $96 - 53 = 43$
- $782 - 531 = 251$
- $632198 - 55421 = 576777$
- $7.9 - 3.7 = 4.2$
- $77.365 - 52.92 = 24.445$
- $30621.5 - 7333.71 = 23287.79$

Multiplying numbers

- $55 \times 19 = 1045$
- $621 \times 78 = 48438$
- $8.9 \times 10 = 89$
- $5.5 \times 1.5 = 8.25$
- $63.3 \times 11.3 = 715.29$

Dividing numbers (rounded to two decimal places)

- $94 \div 6 = 15.67$
- $194 \div 26 = 7.46$
- $1073 \div 11 = 97.55$
- $10.1 \div 3.2 = 3.16$
- $8.99 \div 7.4 = 1.21$

Answers to jokes

- Why was the snake so good at numeracy? He was an Adder
- What tools do you need for numeracy? Multipliers
- Why is arithmetic hard work? Because of all those numbers you have to carry

Tommy's insensible loss = 165 mL

Type of dehydration = hyponatraemic

Estimated weight = 12 kg

Daily fluid requirements (maintenance) = 1090 mL

Extra fluids required to correct deficit = 590 mL

Hourly fluid rates and drop rates

- 112.5 mL/hr and a drop rate of 28.2 drops/min
- 125 mL/hr and a drop rate of 41.6 drops/min

CHAPTER 4 Advancing onwards: taking the whole number apart

Estimated weight for Edward: Edward should weigh 7 kg at 5 months of age.

Feed requirements for Edward are: 1050 mL per 24 hours (estimated) and 945 mL per 24 hours (actual weight).

Shaded areas on fraction diagrams: 2/3 and 1/4

Turning fractions into decimals:

5/8 = 0.625

15/40 = 3/8 = 0.375

5/6 = 0.83·

7/9 = 0.7·

28/96 = 14/48 = 7/24 = 0.2916·

Rounding decimals:

175.33333 (round to one decimal place) = 175.3

7.7689 (round to two decimal places) = 7.77

125.9534 (round to 3 decimal places) = 125.953

Who invented fractions? Henry the ⅛th

BMI and category:

Nathan's BMI = 24.8 kg/m^2

This fits into 'normal' range on adult chart and into 'obesity' in the child growth chart, which, whilst it may be obvious, does illustrate that we should be using child reference data sets at all times and with respect to all areas of children's nursing care and practice (if these are available).

Calculating percentages of whole numbers:

- 53% of 625 = 331.25
- 75% of 95 = 71.25

- 31% of 350 = 108.5
- 12% of 500 = 60

It is worth estimating first before doing the actual calculation, that is, for 53% of 625 work out 50% first = 312.5. This then allows you to check if your answer is correct.

Weight loss in first 2 weeks of life:

- Edward = birth weight 3.5 kg = 350 grams lost in first 2 weeks
- Nathan = birth weight 4.1 kg = 410 grams lost in first 2 weeks

Percentages and solutions

- 250 mL of 5% w/v glucose solution = 5 grams of glucose in 100 mL = 12.5 g of glucose in 250 mL
- 10 mL of 15% w/v potassium chloride = 15 grams of potassium chloride in 100 mL = 1.5 g in 10 mL

Volumes of Magic Medicine A:

7.5 g of Magic Medicine A = 50 mL

22.5 g of Magic Medicine A = 150 mL

45 g of Magic Medicine A = 300 mL

Maintenance fluids

Nathan weighs 42.5 kg so maintenance fluids will be 1000 mL for first 10 kg, 500 mL for next 10 kg and 20 × 22.5 kg for the remainder = 1000 + 500 + 450 = 1950.

The hourly rate will be 1950 ÷ 24 = 81.25 mL per hour.

60% of total daily maintenance fluids and hourly rate = 60/100 × 1950 = 1170 mL in 24 hours and 48.75 mL per hour.

75% of total daily maintenance fluids and hourly rate = 75/100 × 1950 =

1462.5 mL in 24 hours and 60.9 mL per hour.

Results of investigations in percentages:
One example is when measuring the white blood cell count and differential (as part of a full blood count), that is, from a total white cell count of 4.5–12 × 10⁹/L: Neutrophils 40–60%; Lymphocytes 20–40%; Monocytes 2–8%; Eosinophils 1–4%; Basophils 0.5–1% and Band (immature neutrophil) 0–5% (the proportions of one other do vary in parameter dependent on source used). The percentage measurement is also used when monitoring HbA1c, which is explained and covered in more detail in Chapter 7.

Magic potions ratio calculations:

A:B = 10:20 (or 1:2) B:C = 20:5 (or 4:1) C:A = 5:10 (or 1:2)

The amounts needed to make 87.5 mL is 2½ times the amount so A = 25 mL, B = 50 mL and C = 12.5, which you check by adding up to together to make a total of 87.5 mL.

Calculating mg per mL for percentage solutions of lidocaine:

Lidocaine	mg per mL
0.1%	1
0.2%	2
0.5%	5
1%	10
2%	20
5%	50

Converting kcal to kJ and MJ:

Age/ weight	kcal/ kg/day	kJ/kg/ day	MJ/kg/ day
0–6 months	100–110	418.40–460.24	0.4184–0.46
6–12 months	100	418.4	0.4184
10–20 kg	50	209.2	0.2092
>20 kg	20	83.6	0.0836

Edward's energy requirements: 700–770 kcal/day OR 2928.8 kJ/day OR 2.93 mJ/day

CHAPTER 5 Putting the pieces together – a formula for children's nurses

What is a forum? Two –um plus two –um

It is also a public square or market place in an ancient Roma city which was the assembly place for judicial activity and public business. In this day and age we use the term to signify a public meeting place where usually special interests are represented, that is, the forums that form part of the Royal College of Nursing many of which have a special focus on children and young people.

Medicine calculation practice questions:

1. Alice's paracetamol dose in millilitres = 3.8 mL.

   It should not be given till 17.40. She has only had one dose in the day (which was her first one in the last 24 hours) so has not exceeded her maximum daily dose.

2. The dose of co-amoxiclav in millilitres = 6.3 mL and she has been prescribed a correct dose to be able to draw it up accurately (the absolutely correct dose would be 378 mg).

Dose of cefotaxime in millilitres = 6.6 mL (rounded up to one decimal place).

It is the correct dosage though it would be preferable to write it up as 625 mg so as to be able to draw it up accurately as 6.5 mL (rounding down rather than rounding up).

3. It is important to either adjust the amount of diluents (as per pharmacy guidelines and advice) or the prescribed dose to ensure that you can draw up the correct amount without rounding up or down. This is particularly important when working with very small babies as will be discussed in the next chapter where we need to give accurate and therapeutic doses.

4.

Analgesic	Action	Dose	How much for Luke?	Dose supplied in	Dose given
Paracetamol	Non-opioid, analgesic commonly used in children's nursing practice to treat mild to moderate pain and pyrexia	20 mg/kg for severe pain for 48 hours only	540 mg	250 mg in 5 mL	10.8 mL
Ibuprofen	Non-steroidal anti-inflammatory analgesic for mild to moderate pain	30 mg/kg in 3–4 divided doses	270 mg t.d.s. 202.5 mg q.d.s.	100 mg in 5 mL suspension	13.5 mL 10.15 mL

(continued)

Analgesic	Action	Dose	How much for Luke?	Dose supplied in	Dose given
Diclofenac sodium	Non-steroidal anti inflammatory analgesic for mild to moderate pain	0.5–1 mg/kg (max 50 mg) 3 times daily	Calculate a 0.5 mg/kg dose = 13.5 mg	25 mg/50 mg dispersible tablets dissolved in 5 mL of water	2.7 mL
Codeine phosphate	An opioid analgesic used to treat mild to moderate pain	0.5–1 mg/kg every 4–6 hours (max 240 mg daily)	Calculate a 0.8 mg/kg = 21.6 mg	25 mg in 5 mL	4.3 mL
Morphine	An opioid analgesic used to manage moderate to severe pain.	200–500 micrograms/kg (max 20 mg) every 4 hours titrated to response	Calculate a 300 microgram/kg dose = 8.1 mg	Oral solution supplied in 10 mg/5 mL NB – if the solution is above 13 mg/5 mL it becomes a CD	4.1 mL

5.

Weight (if needed)	Medicine	Amount	Route	Frequency	Numeracy problem to be solved	Answer
	Chlorpheniramine	1 mg	Oral	t.d.s.	Supplied in an oral liquid 2 mg in 5 mL. How much will you give?	2.5 mL

	Diazepam	2.5 mg	Oral	Single dose	Supplied in an oral liquid 2 mg in 5 mL. How much will you give?	6.25 mL
13.5 kg	Alfacalcidol	400 nanograms	Oral	Daily	2 micrograms per mL	0.2 mL
12 kg	Cefalexin	30 mg/kg/day	Oral	q.d.s.	Calculate the single dose to be given	90 mg
36 kg	Flucloxacillin	100 mg/kg/day	Oral	q.d.s.	Calculate the single dose to be given	900 mg
	Amoxicillin	160 mg	IV	t.d.s.	The antibiotic is made up so that you have 100 mg/mL. How much will be given?	1.6 mL
	Amoxicillin	160 mg	IV	t.d.s.	The antibiotic is made up so that you have 250 mg/mL. How much will be given?	0.64 mL

CHAPTER 6 Administering medicines and managing numbers in more complex settings – the pharmacist and neonatal nursing perspectives

SI conversions

Kilogram (kg)	Gram (g)	Milligram (mg)	Microgram	Nanogram
0.001	1	1000	1000000	1000000000
0.000006	0.006	6	6000	6000000
0.8	800	800000	800000000	800000000000
0.00000002	0.00002	0.02	20	20000
0.00000025	0.00025	0.25	250	250000
2.75	2750	2750000	2750000000	2750000000000

The etiquette of prescribing

The unnecessary use of decimal points should be avoided – is 3.0 mg correct?
No – it should be prescribed as 3 mg

Quantities of 1 gram or more should be written as 1 g – so if 1500 mg is prescribed how should it be written?
1.5 g

Quantities less than 1 gram should be written in milligrams, that is, 0.5 g =
500 mg

Quantities less than 1 mg should be written in micrograms, that is, 0.75 mg
= **750 micrograms**

When decimals are unavoidable a zero should be written in front of the decimal point where there is no other figure, that is, is .5 mg correct? **NO.** How should it be written? **0.5 mg**

Use of the decimal point is acceptable to express a range, for example, 0.5 to 1 g. **TRUE**

'Micrograms' and 'nanograms' should **not** be abbreviated. Similarly 'units' should **not** be abbreviated. **TRUE**

The term 'millilitre' (mL) is used in medicine and pharmacy, and cubic centimetre, c.c., or cm^3 should not be used. **TRUE**

Source: BNF for Children (2011–2012)

Diluent – how much to add to the following antibiotics:

Amoxicillin 500 mg in a final volume of 5 mL has a displacement value of 0.4 mL = 4.6 mL

Flucloxacillin 250 mg in a final volume of 2.5 mL has a displacement value of 0.2 mL = 2.3 mL

Vancomycin 500 mg in a final volume of 10 mL has a displacement value of 0.3 mL = 9.7 mL

Meropenem 500 mg in a final volume of 5 mL has a displacement value of 0.5 mL = 4.5 mL

Cefotaxime 500 mg in a final volume of 5 mL has a displacement value of 0.2 mL = 4.8 mL

Antibiotic doses for Bobbie

Benzylpenicillin dose = 33.75 mg twice a day

Gentamicin dose = 6.75 mg every 36 hours

Morphine infusions for Bobby

Morphine can come in various strengths from 1 mg/mL, 10 mg/mL, 15 mg/mL, 30 mg/mL and 60 mg/2 mL. What do you think would be the most appropriate strength that should be used in the preparation of the infusion and why? Checking the cost, reducing wastage and ensuring that risk of error reduced by using the amounts most relevant to Bobby who needs 2.7 mg. Using the 1mg/ mL would mean that this equates to 2.7 mL which can then be made up to 20 mL for infusion via pump.

Dopamine infusions

Reduction of 1 microgram/kg/minute. What is the prescribed rate for Bobby? The rate will be reduced by one fifth every four hours so go from 0.25 mL/hr to 0.2 mL per hour for four hours and then 0.15 mL/hr for four hours to be stopped when it gets to 0.1 mL/hr.

Appendix

· ·

FAMOUS MATHEMATICIANS

Numeracy in Children's Nursing, First Edition. Arija Parker

© 2015 John Wiley & Sons, Ltd. Published 2015 by John Wiley & Sons Ltd.

Here is some information on the famous mathematicians that have contributed to the body of knowledge that underpins the basics covered in this book.

Agnesi, Maria (16 May 1718–9 January 1799) wrote the first mathematics book written by a woman and was the first woman to be appointed as mathematics professor in a university. Her book was published in two volumes covering arithmetic, algebra, trigonometry, geometry, calculus, series and differential equations.

Archimedes (circa 287–circa 212 BC) was born in Syracuse in eastern Sicily and was educated in Alexandria in Egypt. His most famous achievements in mathematics included, in mechanics, defining the principle of the lever and for inventing the compound pulley and hydraulic screw for raising water from a lower to higher level. The Archimedes principle states that a body immersed in fluid loses weight equal to the weight of the amount of fluid it displaces. This happened when he was stepping into the bath where apparently he shouted 'Eureka'. Eureka in Halifax (in the United Kingdom) is a museum for children and a great place to visit where you can see this principle in action.

Babbage, Charles (26 December 1791–18 October 1871) was an English mathematician, philosopher, inventor and mechanical engineer who originated the concept of a programmable computer.

Bhaskara is also known as **Bhaskara II** or as **Bhaskaracharya**, which means 'Bhaskara the Teacher'. Bhaskaracharya's father was a Brahmin named Mahesvara, who was famed as an astrologer himself. Bhaskaracharya represented the peak of mathematical knowledge in the 12th century. He reached an understanding of the number systems and solving equations which was not to be achieved in Europe for several centuries. This included an appreciation of the value of zero and negative numbers.

Fibonacci, or more correctly Leonardo da Pisa, was born in Pisa in 1175 AD. In 1200 he returned to Pisa, after travelling widely with his family and used the knowledge he had gained on his travels to write *Liber abaci* in which he introduced the Latin-speaking world to the decimal number system. He also went on to develop the root system and the famous Fibonacci series that is mentioned in the book.

Lovelace, Ada was the daughter of the famous poet, Lord Byron. She was born on 10th December, 1815 in the United Kingdom and is thought to be the 'first programmer' of the world because her mathematical work laid the foundation for the massive world of software and computers. In 1980, the computer programming language 'Ada' was named after her.

Newton, Isaac (1643–1727) was interested in mathematics, optics, physics and astronomy. His greatest work was published in 1687 and showed how a universal force and gravity applied to all objects in all parts of the universe. This is where he is most probably well-known with the story of the apple falling on his head.

Nightingale, Florence (May 12, 1820–August 13, 1910) maybe you would not describe her as a mathematician though some of her statistical work and diagrams would be considered to be such, which is why she is included in this glossary and mentioned in the concluding comments in this book.

Pascal, Blaise (1623–1662) invented the Pascaline, an early calculator. In the 1650s, Pascal laid the foundation of probability theory and published the theological works Pénsees and Provinciales.

Pythagoras (Greek, 570–495 BC) is considered by some to be one of the first great mathematicians. He is also commonly credited with the Pythagorean Theorem within trigonometry. He is considered to be the founding father of modern mathematics.

Turing, Alan Mathison (1912–1954), mathematician and first computer scientist. Invented the Turing test, which is a test of a machine's ability to exhibit intelligent behaviour (artificial intelligence). Considered to be one of the greatest minds of the 20th century with the code breaking work he did during the war with the German Enigma encryptions.

Venn, John Archibald (4 August 1834–4 April 1923), was a British logician and is famous for introducing the Venn diagram, which is used in many fields, including set theory, probability, logic, statistics and computer science.

References

Aldgate J, Jones D, Rose W and Jeffrey C (2006) *The Developing World of the Child*. London: Jessica Kingsley Publishers.

Advanced Life Support Group (2011) *Advanced Paediatric Life Support: The Practical Approach*, 5th edition. Plymouth: BMJ Books/John Wiley & Sons.

Association of Clinical Biochemists (2003) *Guidelines for the Performance of the Sweat Test for the Investigation of Cystic Fibrosis in the UK*. Available at: http://www.acb.org.uk/docs/default-source/committees/scientific/guidelines/acb/sweat-guideline-v2-1.pdf (accessed on 26 March 2015).

Baroody AJ and Ginsburg HP (1990) cited in Gillies R (2004) *Numeracy for Nurses: The Case for Traditional Versus Non-traditional Methods for Teaching Drug Calculations*. Availabe at : http://www.merga.net.au/documents/RP292004.pdf (accessed on 26 March 2015).

Bellos A (2010) *Alex's Adventures in Numberland*. London: Bloomsbury Press.

BNFC (2013) *BNF for Children*. London: BMJ Group, RPS Publishing, RCPCH Publications Ltd.

British Thoracic Society/Scottish Intercollegiate Guidelines Network (2014) *British Guideline on the Management of Asthma A national Clinical guideline*. Edinburgh: SIGN. Available at: https://www.brit-thoracic.org.uk/document-library/clinical-information/asthma/btssign-asthma-guideline-2014/ (accessed on 26 March 2015).

Coben D (2000) Numeracy, mathematics and adult learning. In: Gall (Ed.), *Adult Numeracy Development: Theory, Research, Practice* (pp. 33–50). Cresskill, NJ: HamptonPress.

Collins English Dictionary (1999) *Collins English Dictionary Millennium Edition*, 4th edition. Aylesbury: BCA HarperCollins Publishers.

Dehaene S, Molko N, Cohen L and Wilson AJ (2004) Arithmetic and the brain, *Current Opinion in Neurobiology*, Vol. 14, no. 2, pp. 218–224.

Department for Education (2014) *Statutory Framework for the Early Years Foundation Stage*. Available at: https://www.gov.uk/government/uploads/

Numeracy in Children's Nursing, First Edition. Arija Parker
© 2015 John Wiley & Sons, Ltd. Published 2015 by John Wiley & Sons Ltd.

system/uploads/attachment_data/file/335504/EYFS_framework_from_1_
September_2014__with_clarification_note.pdf (accessed on 26 March 2015).

Enzensburger HM (2000) *The Number Devil: A Mathematical Adventure*, London: Granta Publications.

Galilei G (1623) *Opere II Saggiatore* p. 171.

Goldin G (1990) Epistemology, construction and discovery learning in mathematics. In: Davis RB, Maher C and Noddings N (Eds.), *Journal for Research in Mathematics Education*. Virginia, VA: NCTM.

Hanas R (2010, 2012) *Type 1 Diabetes in Children, Young People and Adults*, 3rd and 4th editions. London: Class Publishing.

Hansman CA (2001) *Context-Based Adult Learning,* In Merriam SB (Ed.) An update on Adult Learning Theory, *New Directions for Adult and Continuing Education*. No. 89, pp. 43–51. San Francisco: Jossey-Bass.

Hutton BM and Gardner H (2005) Calculation skills, *Paediatric Nursing*, Vol. 17, no. 2, pp. 1–19.

Kelly J. (2001) Minimising potential side-effects of medication at different ages, *Professional Nurse*, Vol. 17, no. 4, pp. 259–262.

Kelsey J and McEwing G (Eds.) (2008) *Clinical Skills in Child Health Practice*, London: Churchill Livingstone Elsevier.

Mackway-Jones K, Molyneux E, Phillips B and Wieteska, S (Eds.) (2005) *Advanced Paediatric Life Support – The Practical Approach,* 4th edition, Oxford: BMJ Books, Blackwell publishers.

Modie N (2004) Management of fluid balance in the very immature neonate, *Archives Of Disease In Childhood*, Vol. 89, pp. F108–F111.

Muldoon HC (1916) *Lessons in Pharmaceutical Latin and Prescription Writing and Interpretation*, London: Chapman & Hall. Available at: http://ia700202.us.archive.org/0/items/lessonsinpharmac00mulduoft/lessonsinpharmac00mulduoft.pdf (accessed on 26 March 2015).

National Institute for Health and Clinical Excellence (2004) *Type 1 Diabetes: Diagnosis and Management of Type 1 Diabetes in Children and Young People*. Clinical Guideline 15. London: NICE.

National Institute for Health and Clinical Excellence (2007a) *Acutely Ill Patients in Hospital, Recognition of and Response to Acute Illness in Adults in Hospital*. Clinical Guideline 50. London: NICE.

National Institute for Health and Clinical Excellence (2007b) *Head Injury: Triage, Assessment, Investigation and Early Management of Head Injury in Infants, Children and Adults*. Clinical Guideline 56. London: NICE.

National Institute for Health and Clinical Excellence (2007c) *Feverish Illness in Children*. Clinical Guideline 47. London: NICE.

National Institute for Health and Clinical Excellence (2009) *Diarrhoea and Vomiting in children Diarrhoea and Vomiting Caused by Gastroenteritis: Diagnosis,*

Assessment and Management in Children Younger than 5 Years. NICE Clinical Guideline 84. London: NICE. Available at: http://www.nice.org.uk/guidance/CG84 (accessed on 26 March 2015).

National Patient Safety Agency (2005) *Safer Practice Notice 11: Wristbands for Hospital Inpatients Improve Safety*. Available at: http://www.nrls.npsa.nhs.uk/EasySiteWeb/getresource.axd?AssetID=60032 (accessed on 26 March 2015).

National Patient Safety Agency (2007a) *Safety in Doses Improving the Use of Medicines in the NHS*. Available at: http://www.nrls.npsa.nhs.uk/EasySiteWeb/getresource.axd?AssetID=61626& (accessed on 26 March 2015).

National Patient Safety Agency (2007b) *Further Notice Standardising Wristbands For Patients Improves Patient Safety*. Available at: http://www.nrls.npsa.nhs.uk/resources/?entryid45 = 59824 (accessed on 26 March 2015).

National Patient Safety Agency (2007c) *Reducing the Risk of Hyponatraemia When Administering Intravenous Infusions to Children*. Patient Safety Alert 22. London: NPSA.

Nursing and Midwifery Council (NMC) (2007a) *Standard for Medicine Management*. Available at: http://www.nmc-uk.org/Documents/NMC-Publications/NMC-Standards-for-medicines-management.pdf (accessed on 26 March 2015).

Nursing and Midwifery Council (2007b) *Essential Skills Clusters (ESC's) for Pre-registration Nursing Programmes*. Annexe to NMC Circular 07/2007. London: NMC.

Nursing and Midwifery Council (2010) *Standards for Pre-registration Nursing Education*. London: NMC.

Nursing and Midwifery Council (2015) *The Code Professional standards of practice and behaviour for nurses and midwives*, available at http://www.nmc.org.uk/globalassets/sitedocuments/nmc-publications/revised-new-nmc-code.pdf (accessed 16 June 2015)

Piaget J (1953) *The Origin of Intelligence in the Child*. London and New York: Routledge.

Pozehl BJ (1996) Mathematical calculation ability and mathematical anxiety of baccalaureate nursing students, *Journal of Nursing Education*, Vol. 235, no. 1, pp. 37–39.

Resuscitation Council Available at: http://www.resus.org.uk/siteindx.htm (accessed on 26 March 2015).

Rothman RL, Montori VM, Cherrinton A and Pignone MP (2008) Perspective: the role of numeracy in health care, *Journal of Health Communities*, Vol. 13, no. 6, pp. 583–595.

Royal College of Nursing (2006) *Malnutrition. What Nurses Working with Children and Young People Need to Know and Do*. London: RCN.

Royal College of Nursing (2007) *Standards for Assessing, Measuring and Monitoring Vital Signs in Infants, Children and Young People, RCH Guidance for Children's Nurse and Nurses Working with Children and Young People*. London: RCN.

Royal College of Nursing (2009) *Recognition and Assessment of Acute Pain in Children*. Available at: http://www.rcn.org.uk/development/practice/clinicalguidelines/pain (accessed on 26 March 2015).

Royal College of Obstetricians and Gynaecologists (2010) *Antenatal Corticosteroids to Reduce Neonatal Morbidityand Mortality*. Green-top Guideline No. 7. Available at: http://www.rcog.org.uk/womens-health/clinical-guidance/antenatal-corticosteroids-prevent-respiratory-distress-syndrome-gree (accessed on 26 March 2015).

Sharma MC (1993) Place value concept: how children learn it and how to teach it, *The Center For Teaching/Learning of Mathematics*, Vol. 10, nos. 1 & 2, pp. 1–33.

Skinner S (2005) *Understanding Clinical Investigations: A Quick Reference Guide*. London: Baillere Tindall.

Stanford AS, Chambers CT and Craig, KD (2006) The role of developmental factors in predicting young children's use of a self-report scale for Pain, *Pain*, vol. 20, pp. 16–23.

Sousa DA (2007) *How the Brain Learns Mathematics*. Thousand Oaks, CA: Corwin Press.

Tucker A (2001) *Fractions & Units in Everyday Life*. Available at: www.maa.org (accessed on 26 March 2015).

Wong D and Baker C (1988) Pain in children: comparison of assessment scales. *Pediatric Nursing*, Vol. 14, no. 1, pp. 9–17. Available at: http://www.wongbakerfaces.org/ for a copy of the tool (accessed on 26 March 2015).

Bibliography

Basic Skills Agency (2001) *Adult Numeracy core curriculum,*. London: Cambridge Training and Development Limited. Available at: http://www.counton.org/resources/adultcc/pdfs/resource_130.pdf (accessed on 26 March 2015).

Bouch D and Ness C (2007) *Maths4Life Measurement*. London: NRDC.

Coben D (2003) *Adult Numeracy: Review of Research and Related Literature*. London: NRDC.

Davison N (2008) *Numeracy, Clinical Calculations and Basic Statistics*. Trowbridge: Reflect Press.

Department for Education and Employment & Qualifications and Curriculum Authority (1999) *Mathematics The National Curriculum of England*. Available at: http://webarchive.nationalarchives.gov.uk/20101221004558/http:/curriculum.qcda.gov.uk/uploads/Mathematics%201999%20programme%20of%20study_tcm8-12059.pdf (accessed on 26 March 2015).

Department of Health (2004) *Building a Safer NHS for Patients: Improving Medication Safety*. London: HMSO. Available at: http://webarchive.nationalarchives.gov.uk/20130107105354/http:/www.dh.gov.uk/prod_consum_dh/groups/dh_digitalassets/@dh/@en/documents/digitalasset/dh_4084961.pdf (accessed on 26 March 2015).

Department of Health (2010) *Six Years on: Delivering the Diabetes National Service Framework*. London: DH. Available at: http://webarchive.nationalarchives.gov.uk/20130107105354/http://www.dh.gov.uk/prod_consum_dh/groups/dh_digitalassets/@dh/@en/@ps/documents/digitalasset/dh_112511.pdf (accessed on 26 March 2015).

Department of Health Diabetes Policy Team (2007) *Making Every Young Person with Diabetes Matter*. London: DH. Available at: http://www.diabetes.org.uk/documents/reports/makingeveryyoungpersonmatter.pdf (accessed on 26 March 2015).

General Medical Council (2013) *Good Practice in Prescribing Medicines – Guidance for Doctors*. Available at: http://www.gmc-uk.org/guidance/ethical_guidance/prescriptions_faqs.asp(accessed on 26 March 2015). (accessed on 26 March 2015).

Numeracy in Children's Nursing, First Edition. Arija Parker

© 2015 John Wiley & Sons, Ltd. Published 2015 by John Wiley & Sons Ltd.

Gopnik A, Meltzoff A and Kuhl P (1999) *The Scientist in the Crib: Minds, Brains and How Children Learn*, Fairfield, NJ: William Morrow and Company.

Haylock D and Cockburn A (2008) *Understanding Mathematics for Young Children: A Guide for Foundation Stage & Lower Primary Teachers.* London: Sage Publications Ltd.

Hutton M (2009) *Essential Calculation Skills for Nurses, Midwives and Healthcare Practitioners.* Maidenhead: Open University Press.

Kanneh A (2002a) Paediatric pharmacological principles: an update, Part 1: Drug development and pharmacodynamics. *Paediatric Nursing*, vol.14, no. 8, pp. 36–42.

Kanneh A (2002b) Paediatric pharmacological principles: an update, Part 2: Pharmacokinetics: absorption and distribution. *Paediatric Nursing*, vol.14, no. 9, pp. 39–43.

Kanneh A (2002c) Paediatric pharmacological principles: an update, Part 3: Pharmacokinetics: metabolism and excretion. *Paediatric Nursing*, vol.14, no. 10, pp. 36–43.

Kanneh A. (2004) Adverse drug reactions in children: Part 1. *Paediatric Nursing*, vol. 16, no. 6, pp. 32–35.

Large T (2006) *The Usborne Illustrated Dictionary of Maths: With Recommended Websites.* London: Usborne Publishing Limited.

London Strategic Unit (2007) *Embedded Literacy, Language and Numeracy.* London: Institute of Education.

McLeod R and Newmarch B (2006) *Fractions, Maths4Life.* London: NRDC.

Moon J (1999) *Reflection in Learning and Professional Development.* London: Kogan Page.

Mulholland JM (2007) *The Nurse, The Math, The Meds: Drug Calculations Using Dimensional Analysis.* St Louis, MI: Mosby Elsevier.

O'Connor JJ and Robertson EF (2000) *History Topic: A History of Zero*, Available at: http://www-history.mcs.st-andrews.ac.uk/HistTopics/Zero.html(accessed on 26 March 2015).

Swain J, Baker E, Holder D, Newmarch B and Coben D (2005) *Beyond the Daily Application: Making Numeracy Teaching Meaningful to Adult Learners.* London: NRDC.

Watt S (2003a) Safe administration of medicines to children: part 1. *Paediatric Nursing*, vol. 15, no. 4, pp. 40–43.

Watt S (2003) Safe administration of medicines to children: part 2, *Paediatric Nursing*, vol. 15, no. 5, pp. 40–44.

Wilcock J and Jewkes F (2000) Making sense of fluid balance in children. *Paediatric Nursing,* vol. 12, no. 7, pp. 37–42.

Williams JDP (2007) Medication errors. *Journal of the Royal College of Physicians*, vol. 37, pp. 343–346.

Index

absorption of drugs 141–2
accuracy 31
acid–base balance 217
addition 69–71
    fractions 106–7
ADME memory aid 142
administration errors 5, 170
    reducing 171–3
adolescent development 218
adrenaline 121–2
alfacalcidol 158
alkalaemia 217
alkalosis 217
amoxicillin 153, 159
anaesthetics, local 119
analgesics 156–7
angles 48
Apgar score 165–7
Arch Mede Faces Pain Scale 23
arterial blood gases 217–18
associative operations 69–70
asthma 62
augmentin 153
auscultation 35
AVPU tool for neurological
    assessment 59

basal metabolic rate (BMR) 125–6
bases of numbers 15–17

basophils 134
Beer–Lambert law 58
blood
    arterial gases 217–18
    white cells 134–5
blood glucose monitoring 197,
    209, 216
blood pressure 50–53
BoDMAS/BiDMAS memory aid 82–3
body mass index (BMI) 113–14
body surface area (BSA) 47–8, 86

calculators, use of 32, 86–87
capillary refill time (CRT) 57, 92
carbohydrate intake monitoring 198
cardinal numbers 12
cardinal principle 205
cefalexin 159
cefotaxime 153–4
Celsius temperature scale 49–50
child growth and development
    122, 200
    adolescence 218
    definition 201
    early adulthood 219–20
    energy requirements 126
    Key Stage 1 (KS1) 211–13
    Key Stage 2 (KS2) 213–14
    Key Stage 3 (KS3) 218–19

Numeracy in Children's Nursing, First Edition. Arija Parker
© 2015 John Wiley & Sons, Ltd. Published 2015 by John Wiley & Sons Ltd.

child growth and development (*Cont.*)
    middle childhood development
        210–11
    milestones 201–3
    numerical skills 203
    preschool development 203–7
chlorpheniramine 158
clavulanic acid 153
clocks, 12-hour or 24-hour 37–8
co-amoxiclav 153
codeine phosphate 156
commutative operations 70
conceptual errors 21
converting measurement
        units 39–40
    weight 44
counting 32–3
    playing with children 33
    pulse or heart rate 36
    respirations 34–5
    time 36–8
C-reactive protein (CRP) 135
cuff sizes for sphygmomanometers 53
cystic fibrosis (CF) 123–4

decilitre, definition 16
decimal numbers 108–9
    rounding 109
decimal points 71, 171
defective procedure/method errors 21
dehydration
    estimating percentage
        dehydration 93
    management of mild dehydration
        93–4
diabetes insipidus 196
diabetes mellitus, type 1
    advice to parents 210
    blood glucose monitoring 197
    carbohydrate intake monitoring 198
    definition 195–6

exercise 200
    glycaemic index (GI) 199–200
    HbA1c monitoring 197–8
    insulin administration 196–7
    key principles 196–200
    middle childhood 214–16
    at two years old 208–9
    urine testing 198
diabetic ketoacidosis (DKA) 193,
        216–17
diastole 50–51
diastolic blood pressure 50–51
diazepam 158
diclofenac sodium 156
digits 17
dispensing errors 5, 170
    reducing 171
displacement values 178
distribution of drugs 142
division 80–82
    fractions 107–8
dopamine 185–7
dosage calculations 151–9
drug reconstitution 173–4
dyscalculia 6
    definition 10–11
dyslexia 10–11
dyspraxia 10–11

Eatwell plate 109–11
electrolytes 67
energy intake 125
energy requirements for growth and
        development 126
eosinophils 135
equivalent fractions 104–5
errors in medical practice 5
errors in numeracy practice 21–2
    conceptual errors 21
    defective procedure/method
        errors 21

overgeneralisation errors 21
random response errors 21
undergeneralisation errors 21
vocabulary errors 21
wrong operation errors 21
erythrocyte sedimentation rate (ESR) 135
excretion of drugs 142
exercise and diabetes 200
extracellular fluid (ECF) 84–5

factors 81
Fahrenheit temperature scale 49–50
failure to thrive 99–100
fever 86
Fibonacci series 19–20
flow rates, calculating 94–5
flucloxacillin 159
fluid balance 83–5
    assessing hydration 90–91
    calculating flow rates 94–5
    calculating fluid deficit 92–3
    capillary refill time (CRT) 92
    charts 67
    estimating percentage
        dehydration 93
    estimating weight 91
    management of mild dehydration
        93–4
    positive and negative balances
        85–9
    worked example 88–9
fluid management 119–21, 180–182
formula 148–53
fraction of inspired oxygen (FiO$_2$)
    57, 187
fractions 103–6
    adding and subtracting 106–7
    equivalent fractions 104–5
    language of 113
    multiplying and dividing 107–8

nursing practice examples
    109–14
vulgar fractions 105
full blood count (FBC) 3

gas volumes 42–3
gastroenteritis 85
gene inheritance 123–4
gentamicin 171–2
glucose 84, 118
glycaemic index (GI) 199–200

half-life of drugs 143
head measurement 41–2
heart rate, counting 36
homeostasis 84
hydration, assessing 90–91
hypernatraemic dehydration 90
hypoglycaemia 197
hyponatraemic dehydration 90
hypovolaemic shock 85

ibuprofen 156
ILCOR/ALSG emergency quick weight
    calculation 45
imperial units for weight 45–6
infinity, definition 20
infusions 185–7
inheritance 123–4
insensible loss 86–8
insulin
    administration 196–7
    dosage 208–9, 215
    units 16, 197–8
intercellular fluid (ICF) 84–5
interstitial fluid (ISF) 84
intravascular fluid (IVF) 84
intravenous medication 177–8
isotonic dehydration 90

joule, unit of energy 125

ketoacidosis 118
Korotkoff sounds 52

language of numeracy
    mathematics versus numeracy 11–12
    numbers 12
Latin, use of 147
learning theories 11
leukocytes 134
    basophils 134
    eosinophils 135
    lymphocytes 134
    monocytes 134
    neutrophils 134
lidocaine 119
local anaesthetics 119
lymphocytes 134

malnutrition 127–8
mathematicians, famous 238–9
mathematics see also numeracy
    definition 12
    formula 148–53
    numeracy versus mathematics
        11–12
    teaching in schools 8
mean airway pressure (MAP) 187
measurement
    blood pressure 50–53
    converting units 39–40, 44
    head dimensions 41–2
    pain assessment 53
    pressure 50–53
    SI units 38–47
    surface area 47–8, 86
    temperature 48–50
    volume 42–3
    weight 43–6
medication errors 5
mega, definition 39
metabolism of drugs 142

micro, definition 39
milli, definition 39
modified GCS tool for neurological
        assessment 59–60
mole, unit of chemical amount 181–2
molecular weights 181–2
monocytes 134
morphine 156
    calculating requirements 182–5
multiplication 74–80
    fractions 107–8

nano, definition 39
negative numbers 89
neonatal care 165
    Apgar score 165–7
    dilution fluid 176–7
    displacement values 178
    dopamine requirements 185–7
    errors 170–173
    fluid requirements 179
    intravenous medication 177–8
    maintenance fluid 176
    morphine requirements 182–5
    nurse, role of 169–70
    nursing perspectives 173–5
    off-label/not licensed
        medicines 173
    pharmacist, role of 167–9, 173
    practicalities involving numbers
        175–7
    ventilation 187–8
neurological assessment 58–60
    AVPU tool 59
    modified GCS tool 59–60
neutrophils 134
NHS memory aid 149
Nightingale, Florence 224–5, 239
nominal numbers 13
not licensed for neonatal use
        medicines 173

number lines 89
numbers
  bases of numbers 15–17
  cardinal numbers 12
  decimal numbers 108–9
  definition 12
  digits 17
  Fibonacci series 19–20
  fractions 103–8
  negative numbers 89
  nominal numbers 13
  ordinal numbers 13
  patterns in numbers 19–21
  percentages 114–21
  place values 13–15, 17–18, 70
  positive numbers 89
  powers of numbers 15
  prime numbers 18–19
  proportions 123
  ratio 121–2
  rounding 109
  square roots 86–7
  whole numbers 32–3
  zero as a number and placeholder
    17–18
numeracy
  assessment of 6–7, 30–31, 69,
    102–3, 138–9
  definition 9
  errors 21–2
  language of 11–21
  teaching 7–9
  using skills 223–6
numerals 12
numerical operations
  addition 69–71
  associative operations 69–70
  BoDMAS/BiDMAS memory
    aid 82–3
  commutative operations 70
  division 80–82

  multiplication 74–80
  order of 82–3
  subtraction 71–3

obesity 100–101
off-label medicines 173
oral rehydration solution (ORS) 93–4
ordinal numbers 13
osmotic pull 90
overgeneralisation errors 21
oxygen
  administration 61
  fraction of inspired oxygen (FiO_2)
    57, 187
  oxygen saturation 57–8

Paediatric Early Warning Scores
    (PEWS) 54
  capillary refill time (CRT) 57
  charts 55–6
  definition 54–7
  fraction of inspired oxygen
    (FiO_2) 57
  neurological assessment 58–60
  oxygen saturation 57–8
  record keeping 57
  trigger scores 56
pain assessment in children 23, 53
  tools 23–5
paracetamol 151–2, 156
pascal, unit of pressure 50
patterns in numbers 19–21
peak expiratory flow rate (PEFR) 62
peak inspiratory pressure (PIP) 187
percentage dehydration 93
percentages 114–15
  converting to a decimal 116–17
  converting to a fraction 115
  nursing practice examples 117–21
Periodic Table of Elements 181–2
pH scale 217

pharmacists 167–9, 173
pharmacology 139–40
  absorption 141–2
  distribution 142
  excretion 142
  half-life of drugs 143
  metabolism 142
  pharmacodynamics 140–141
  pharmacokinetics 140
  prescription charts 143–4, 145–7,
    169
  'rights' of medicine administration
    144–5
pi 48
Piaget, Jean 202–3, 204, 205–6,
  211, 219
place values of numbers 13–15,
  17–18, 70
plasma proteins 84–5
positive end expiratory pressure (PEEP)
  187
positive numbers 89
potassium 85
pounds-and-ounces weighing system
  45–6
powers of numbers 15
prefixes for units 39
preschool child development 203–7
prescribing errors 5, 170
prescription charts 143–7, 169
pressurised metered-dose inhalers
  (PMDIs) 33–4, 42–3
prime numbers 18–19
probability 123–4
proportions 123
pulse rate, counting 36
pupil size chart 60

random response errors 21
ratio 121
  nursing practice examples 121–2

reconstitution of drugs 173–4
respirations, counting 34–5
Resuscitation Council emergency quick
    weight calculation 45
'rights' of medicine administration
    144–5
rounding numbers 109

schemata 204
SI units 38–40
  converting units 39–40, 44
  mole 181–2
  volume 42–3
  weight 43–6
social context of learning 11
sodium 84–5, 90
solutes 84
solutions 117–18
sphygmomanometers 50, 52–3
square roots 86–7
steroids 162–3
stones-and-pounds weighing system
    45–6
subtraction 71–3
  fractions 106–7
surface area 47–8, 86
surfactants 167
symbols 48
syringes 155–6
systole 50–51
systolic blood pressure 50–51

teaching numeracy 7–9
temperature 48–9
  Fahrenheit and Celsius scales
    49–50
thermometers 48–9
time 36–7, 48
  12-hour or 24-hour clocks 37–8
  units of time measurement 37
total parenteral nutrition (TPN) 176

umbilical arterial catheter (UAC) 163
undergeneralisation errors 21
urea 67
urine output 179–80
urine testing 198
using numeracy skills 223–6

vancomycin 174
ventilation 187–8
Venturi masks 61
vital sign monitoring 34
   blood pressure 50–53
   counting pulse or heart rate 36
   counting respirations 34–5
   frequency 60
   pain assessment 53
   temperature 48–50
   weight 43–6
vocabulary errors 21

volume, units of 42–3
vulgar fractions 105

weight
   emergency quick calculation
     45, 91
   units of 43–6
white blood cells 134
   basophils 134
   eosinophils 135
   lymphocytes 134
   monocytes 134
   neutrophils 134
whole numbers 32–3
wristbands 31–2
wrong operation errors 21

zero as a number and placeholder
   17–18